ROYAL NAVY
SEARCH AND RESCUE
A CENTENARY CELEBRATION

David Morris AMA
Curator of Aircraft,
Fleet Air Arm Museum

AMBERLEY

Dedicated to those who were not in peril, but who set out to assist others that were.

Cover Image: (MOD Crown Copyright 2014)

First published 2015

Amberley Publishing
The Hill, Stroud
Gloucestershire, GL5 4EP

www.amberley-books.com

Copyright © David Morris AMA, 2015

The right of David Morris AMA to be identified as the Author of this work has been asserted in accordance with the Copyrights, Designs and Patents Act 1988.

ISBN 978 1 4456 3463 0 (paperback)
ISBN 978 1 4456 3474 6 (ebook)

British Library Cataloguing in Publication Data.
A catalogue record for this book is available from the British Library.

Typeset in 11pt on 13pt Sabon LT Std.
Typesetting by Amberley Publishing.
Printed in the UK.

CONTENTS

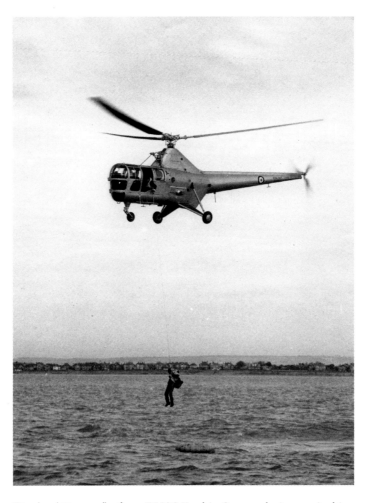

Westland Dragonfly, from RNAS Ford in Sussex, during a winching exercise. (FAA Museum)

FOREWORD

By Captain Eric Brown CBE, DSC, AFC Hon. FRAeS, RN: David Morris, the author of this short but splendid book, has for sixteen years been the Curator of Aircraft at the Fleet Air Arm Museum at Yeovilton, Somerset, so is well versed in naval aircraft.

He chose the subject of Royal Navy Search and Rescue because this usually occurs over open sea, which can be cruel and more treacherous than any other natural environment, and therefore demands aircrew of iron will and stout courage to meet its challenges.

David traces the early beginnings of SAR, when limitations in appropriate equipment severely constrained the capabilities of this vital service, until the helicopter appeared on the scene and was developed rapidly by the military to expand its performance and load-carrying to a remarkable degree.

He describes some difficult SAR episodes to whet the reader's appetite for cliff-hanger flying, leading him to such gripping rescues that he will surely finish up in his armchair with white knuckles clasped around the arms.

This is a well-researched book and a most welcome tribute to the early pioneers of Royal Navy SAR as well as the magnificently professional crews of today, for, make no mistake, this is a team game like no other in the world.

Eric Brown

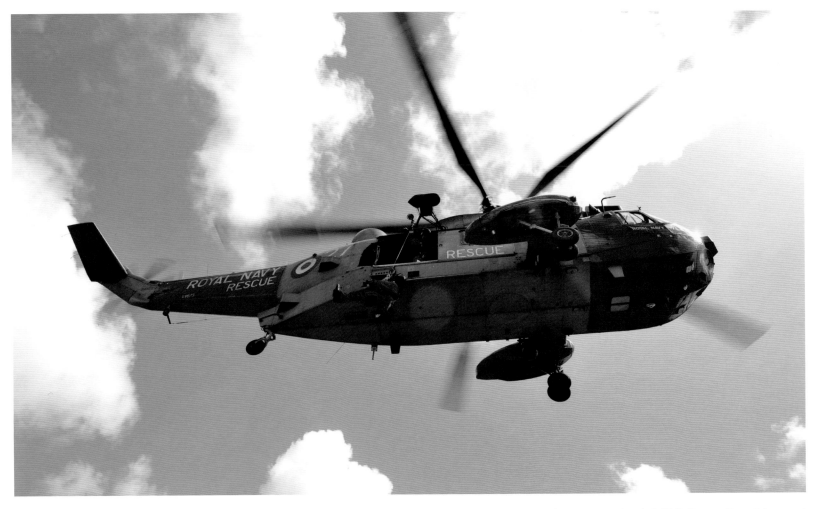

A view that many a stranded sailor or mountaineer would be very pleased to see, a Royal Navy SAR helicopter hovering overhead. (MOD Crown Copyright 2014)

INTRODUCTION: 'SCRAMBLE THE SAR' – 100 YEARS OF ROYAL NAVY SEARCH AND RESCUE

The first time that man set out to locate and bring back to safety a lost friend, animal or precious object, the concept of Search and Rescue was born. Over the thousands of years since, the ability, success rate and level of equipment used to accomplish this has improved dramatically. From searching on foot to today's satellite navigation methods, man has constantly strived to send aid and preserve life if there is still the remotest chance of being able to do so.

Today, the sight of a helicopter speeding toward some destination is familiar enough, but take a moment to consider; is there a life at stake? Is someone in peril and on a knife edge of survival, and will the helicopter crew be selflessly placing themselves in the most dangerous of situations for the sake of saving others?

1

SEARCH AND RESCUE, AIR SEA RESCUE

The phrases 'Search and Rescue' and 'Air Sea Rescue' can be the same thing, but are technically two different disciplines. Many purely coastal-based organisations such as the Coast Guard Service or oil rig helicopter operators usually restrict their flying to coastal and maritime duties, providing only Air Sea Rescue support. However, services such as the Royal Navy and the Royal Air Force can respond to emergency calls in all locations, whether it is sea or land, making them all-encompassing Search and Rescue 'SAR' units.

Royal Navy pilots and observers (navigators) make particularly competent SAR crews as their normal operational flying demands extremely high levels of skill and adaptability every time they take off and fly.

Low-level flying at sea is deceptively dangerous, and operating from ships even more so. Visibility can change from clear blue skies to thick fogs and heavy rain in minutes. They may take off from a ship in fine weather, but return to find their ship (their only landing site) swathed in mist. There is no other option; they just have to be ready for it and ready to adapt and switch to poor weather condition flying in an instant. Few people appreciate just how dangerous this really is. The ship will often be moving forwards and may well be pitching and rolling. Getting closer, the danger level increases as the pilot has to be aware not only of the ship's movements, but also aerial masts, cranes, superstructure and any other aircraft or personnel on what is often a wet and slippery deck.

Poor weather conditions at sea can merge the sky and sea into one flat grey seamless sheet, with no horizon, no up, no down and no clear distinction between sky and water. This makes competent instrument flying an essential skill for all Navy pilots. The term given to this is 'blind flying', and a pilot will have to be able to switch instantly from clear view flying to instruments only (blind flying) if he encounters rain, fog or a low cloud bank. They cannot pull over and wait, or park up and think about it, they just have to be able to do it as second nature for the sake of their crew, passengers and the aircraft.

Of equal importance is the observer, or navigator, often overlooked as a vital component of this team. The observer has as many challenges as the pilot to ensure that the aircraft gets to its destination or target and then, of course, returns safely to base, whether ship or land. Remember, at sea there are no landmarks! No churches, rivers, roads, towns or motorways to check your route against. The observer has to be totally focussed on plotting the course and staying aware of the aircraft's position and (if flying from a ship) the ship's position at all times. Monitoring flight time, distance covered, fuel use and amount of fuel required to return to base (or ship) are all part of the observer's role. Helicopters can only carry a limited fuel load and so calculating the amount they will need and use on a flight is critical. This becomes even more important during a flight where hovering over a target area is involved, as helicopters use considerably more fuel when hovering than in ordinary level flight. SAR missions will frequently require the helicopter to hover while rescuing a stranded person (or persons) and this, by the nature of the task, will be at the furthest extent of the flight. The pilot will have his mind totally focussed on flying the aircraft and will be relying on the observer to be monitoring the fuel and counting down as to when they have to leave the target area and return to base. Of course, the observer must also be aware of the flight plan, plotting the weather, other air traffic and shipping, as well as communicating with air traffic controllers and other ships and aircraft.

If the rescue mission is part of a military operation in hostile waters, the ship from which they departed will keep moving and likely alter course in case it too was being watched by the enemy. This will have been pre-arranged immediately before take off and it will be the observer's responsibility to navigate the helicopter across the featureless sea to the rescue point and then navigate safely back to a different point, i.e. where the ship will now be, not where it previously was. In a live combat situation, this may have to be achieved successfully under radio silence.

You may be imagining all of this happening in daylight, but remember this may also have to be accomplished at night, in extreme weather and, if in combat, perhaps under enemy fire. Both pilot and observer depend on each other totally and develop very strong working bonds, knowing exactly how the other thinks and responds in difficult and critical situations.

Since the introduction of fixed-wing aircraft into the Royal Navy in 1911, its flying duties have never been restricted purely to operations at sea. Royal Naval Air Service (RNAS) units have operated aircraft from land-based airfields or between land bases and ships from the First World War to the present day. The Royal Navy has provided aircraft support for Royal Marine Commando operations worldwide and operated both individually and alongside the RAF and the Army in many combat or humanitarian aid situations globally for over 100 years.

This history of versatile and demanding flying is what enables Royal Navy aircrews to perform so well in search and rescue tasks, enabling them to cope with not just varying sea conditions but also extreme mountain, arctic, desert or jungle conditions if such a rescue operation is required.

Many assume that when a rescue aircraft has arrived on scene then everything is safe. However, there is still much that can go wrong, with no certain safety until aircraft, crew and rescued party are all safely back at base and on the ground.

2

THE FIRST RESCUE BY AIRCRAFT

The first recorded instance of an aircraft being used to provide emergency assistance must surely be credited to American pioneer aviator Hugh Robinson in August 1911. Using his Curtiss hydro-plane to land on Lake Michigan, Robinson assisted fellow aviator Rene Simon, who had made a forced landing on the water. This extraordinary display of flying skill and bravery demonstrated the potential for aircraft to become versatile platforms for many fast response uses, search and rescue clearly being among them.

The first recognised successful military rescue using an aircraft was carried out by a Royal Naval Air Service pilot during the First World War. On 19 November 1915, Squadron Commander Richard Bell-Davies (later to become Vice-Admiral Sir Richard Bell-Davies VC CB DSO AFC) was operating in command of No. 3 Squadron RNAS on light bombing missions over Ferijik Junction, Bulgaria, close to the Ottoman-controlled European border.

During the raid his fellow airman, Flight Sub-Lieutenant Smylie's aircraft was damaged by ground fire, forcing him down behind enemy lines. He survived the landing but was now in perilous danger as Bulgarian troops raced towards him.

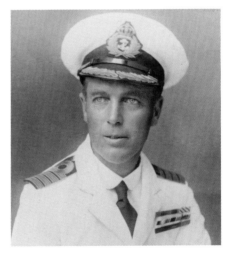 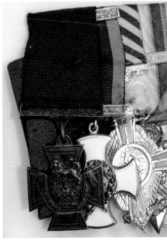

Above left: Richard Bell-Davies was awarded the Victoria Cross for his outstanding bravery and airmanship on 19 November 1915 (medal awarded January 1916). Pictured here as Captain and Head of Naval Air Section in 1920. (FAA Museum)

Above right: Richard Bell-Davies' Victoria Cross in the collection at the Fleet Air Arm Museum, Yeovilton, Somerset. (FAA Museum)

Seeing the sequence of events from his own aerial position, and knowing there was no time to hesitate, Bell-Davies flew his own aircraft down and risked a landing on rough and unprepared ground near his escaping comrade. There was no guarantee that the ground would be suitable for a safe landing, and no knowing if there would be enough clear and obstacle-free space to enable a safe take-off, but Bell-Davies was determined not to leave his fellow pilot stranded and in grave danger.

By luck and skill, he was able to land his Nieuport 12 aircraft close enough to allow Smylie to clamber aboard. However, this was no easy task as the aircraft had been temporarily modified from a two-seat to a single-seat type. This modification entailed covering over the forward seat position, so that access to this position was now only possible through a small gap under the control panel between Bell-Davies' feet. With seconds to spare, Smylie squeezed himself headfirst through the gap and had to crouch on all fours, kneeling on the fuselage frame rails while Bell-Davies took off.

With the Bulgarian troops closing in fast, Bell-Davies managed to negotiate the rough terrain and coax his aircraft back into the air, returning safely to base. Deservedly, Bell-Davies was awarded the Victoria Cross for his actions and the first military rescue using an aircraft had been achieved.

Again during the First World War, an RNAS aircraft crew were involved with an airborne rescue mission with an unusual end to the story. On 5 September 1917, a de Havilland DH-4 fighter bomber and Curtiss H-12 Flying Boat 8666 were patrolling over the North Sea on anti-Zeppelin duties. They engaged two German Zeppelins some 50 miles from the English coast and exchanged gunfire. Both aircraft sustained damage and the DH-4 aircraft lost engine power and had no choice but to make a crash landing in the sea. The Curtiss H-12 crew immediately put down alongside the stricken

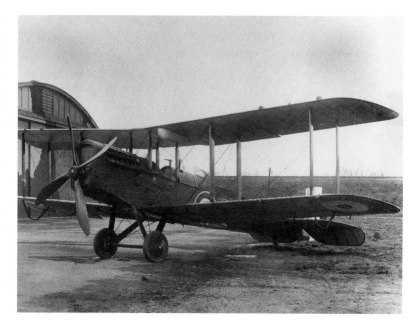

De Havilland type DH4, similar to those used by the RNAS for patrols over the North Sea. (FAA Museum)

DH-4 and rescued the crew into the flying boat. Although they were all safe, the flying boat was now over-loaded for a take-off and the only option was to taxi the flying boat in the direction of their base at Yarmouth. This may sound straightforward, but controlling a lumbering flying boat in the rough conditions of the North Sea is no easy task. After four hours the fuel finally ran out and the aircraft was now left helpless and drifting. Worse still, the hull of the flying boat had been damaged by the German gunfire, was leaking badly, and had to be constantly bailed out.

In an age before effective radio and radar communication, the only long-distance method of delivering a signal back to base was by homing pigeon and most RNAS flying boat crews carried pigeons as a means of sending urgent messages. This may have been the dawn of aviation and modern technology, but in certain circumstances at this time homing pigeons represented a more reliable form of message sending than Morse signals.

The flying boat crew carried four pigeons and released each one at intervals with messages attached giving an approximate location. The fourth of the released pigeons (released on the third day at sea) did make it to Yarmouth and its message formed the basis of a major search operation. Sadly, but miraculously, the body of the first pigeon (released on day one) was found on the beach near Yarmouth that same day, having died from exhaustion while delivering its vital message two days earlier. The information on its attached message provided more details to aid the search. As a result, HMS *Halcyon* located the stricken aircraft and was able to rescue the crew, who were lucky to still be alive after three gruelling days at sea with no food and suffering from exposure and sea sickness.

The body of the first pigeon – known officially as Pigeon No. NURP/17/F/16331 – was preserved and had a place of special honour in the officers' mess at Yarmouth Naval Base, a brass plate reading 'A Very Gallant Gentleman'.

Many lessons in communication and response were learned in these two incidents. Much thought was now given to how aircraft could be made safer for flying at sea, and how aircraft might be used to perform rescues in the future. Technological development after the First World War pushed the development of aircraft forward immensely. The ability to manufacture aluminium sheet in much larger sizes than before opened up many new possibilities and many new, larger aircraft designs began to appear, with float planes and flying boats benefiting greatly from this new technology.

At the end of the First World War, the amalgamation of the Royal Naval Air Service and the Royal Flying Corps into the newly formed Royal Air Force saw the introduction of the first formalised Search and Rescue unit under control of the RAF Marine Craft Section. This newly formed section was to provide

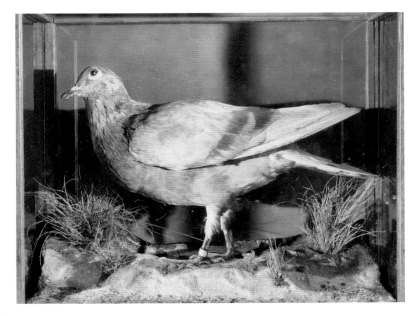

His Majesty's Pigeon No. NURP/17/F/16331, preserved as a mark of respect after its valiant attempt to deliver the vital message in 1918. (RAF Museum Hendon)

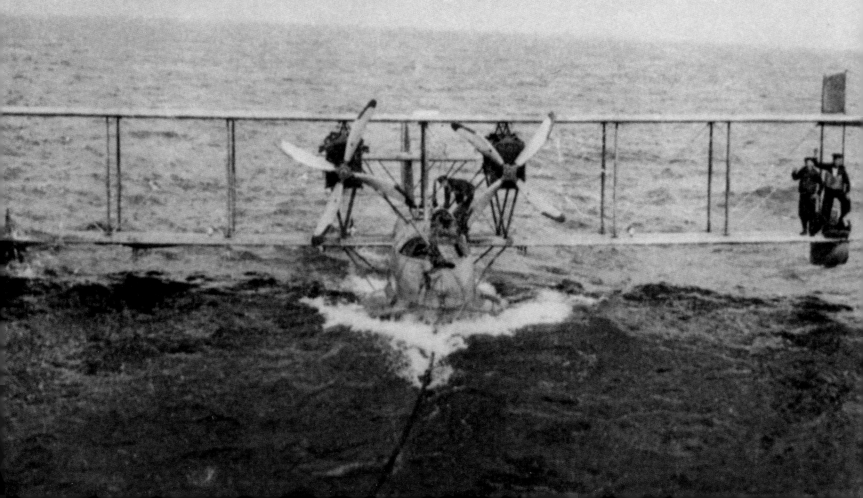

Archive image, believed to be of Curtiss H12 No. 8666 being taken into tow by HMS *Halcyon*. Two ship's crew ratings balance on the outer port wing to counter-balance a damaged starboard side wing tip and float. Wet and very cold, the crew of N8666 had to take turns at doing this for three days and nights to stop the aircraft from sinking. (FAA Museum)

back up for flying boats, its motto being 'The sea shall not have them'. By 1939 the Royal Navy had retaken possession of its flying branch, re-titled the Fleet Air Arm, and henceforth the Royal Navy and RAF have operated their own individual Search and Rescue units and squadrons.

By the 1930s, naval floatplanes such as the Fairey IIIF and IIID, Fairey Sea Fox, Blackburn Shark and Fairey Swordfish were well established types, capable of being used for some rescue and recovery missions if weather and sea conditions permitted. However, being designed to carry a maximum of three people (including the pilot) reduced their effectiveness. As already mentioned, the observer was essential for safe navigation at sea and so picking up a single stranded person was the maximum that could be achieved with such an aircraft. Landing a floatplane in good conditions is relatively straight forward for a skilled, trained pilot, but rough or choppy sea states can make a safe landing and take off with a float plane dangerous, if not impossible, to achieve safely.

Flying boats have more resilience to poor weather and rougher sea conditions than floatplanes, and most are generally capable of carrying a small number of passengers in addition to the crew. The Supermarine Walrus and Sea Otter would prove to be two of the most robust and useful small flying boats in service with both the Fleet Air Arm and RAF. The Walrus entered naval service in 1933 and remained in service until the late 1940s, and the Sea Otter has the honour of being the last biplane to enter service with the Royal Navy, in 1942, remaining in service until the early 1950s and seeing service in the Korean War. True amphibians, these aircraft could operate from airfields or aircraft carriers using their wheeled undercarriage; with their

undercarriage fully retracted, they could perform very capable water landings in conditions considered far too dangerous or marginal for other waterborne aircraft of that time. In addition, they could be carried on a battleship or cruiser, being launched from a turret-mounted catapult platform. On completion of their mission (and if not returning to dry land) they would land alongside the mother ship and be craned back onto the catapult platform ready for a next mission. Such versatility was to mark out both the Walrus and Sea Otter as two of the most notable seaplanes of the era.

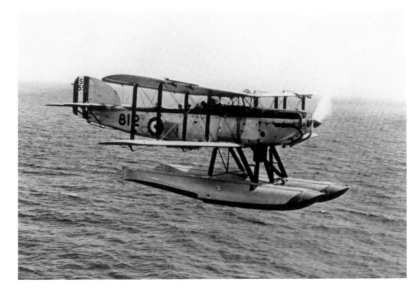

Fairey IIIF, typical of the three-seat float planes used by the Royal Navy during the 1920s and 30s. (FAA Museum)

A sea rescue routine for either Walrus or Otter would ideally see the aircraft land downwind of the target and taxi its way (ideally still into the wind) towards the stranded pilot, who would hopefully be floating in his survival dinghy or life jacket. The wheels of the aircraft could be lowered during this operation to act as temporary drop keels, extending bottom weight to the aircraft and helping to prevent rolling and pitching. This would have to be done by hand (normally by the observer) as the aircraft had no power-operated device to raise or lower the undercarriage, only a basic hand-operated pump. The observer would then crawl to the front of the aircraft and, from the forward hatch, direct operations and guide the pilot in close enough to throw a line to the stranded airman. With the line secured between the airman/dinghy and a horn on the front of the aircraft, the stranded pilot would now (hopefully) float underneath the aircraft wing and alongside the fuselage as the aircraft continued to move forwards, towing the dingy and/or airman through the water. The observer would now clamber back through the fuselage to the rear hatch, where he would be better able to reach the airman in the water and haul him aboard.

With the rescue completed, the dingy would likely be stabbed with a knife and allowed to sink – there would be little time to deflate it and pull it into the aircraft, and it could present a hazard if it became entangled with the aircraft. All the time the aircraft is on the water it is vulnerable to buffeting and being swamped by large waves, striking obstacles or getting water in the engine, so as soon as the rescue was complete the pilot would be anxious to get airborne as swiftly as possible. To enable this, the observer would now clamber back to the front hatch and ensure the rescue rope was gathered in and the hatch closed, clamber back to the

centre section and raise the undercarriage, then strap himself in for take off or tend to the rescued airman if he was injured. Difficult enough under practice conditions, doing this for real in a heavy sea is a dangerous and demanding sequence of events. Keeping the fuselage hatches open for the absolute minimum of time was critical in heavy seas and the whole operation was open to enormous scope for errors and catastrophe, particularly if the person to be rescued were injured, unconscious (or dead) or unable to assist with getting into the aircraft.

One extraordinary rescue mission utilising the Walrus is particularly worthy of note. In January 1941, the merchant ship SS *Eumaeus* was torpedoed by an Italian submarine approximately 100 miles off the West African coast, while transporting British troops. On receiving the signal of the attack, Royal Marine pilot Lt V. B. G. Cheesman launched his Walrus seaplane at 7 a.m. from Freetown harbour and headed out to the stricken vessel. Arriving over the area he found the SS *Eumaeus* to be sunk, leaving dozens of men bobbing around in the cold, shark-infested waters and clinging to any scraps of debris that they could for their survival.

What could he do? There were far more survivors than he could pick up in his aircraft. While Cheesman and his crew were assessing the situation, they flew low and threw out their own inflatable dinghy to a group of the survivors. If nothing else, the men in the water would know they had been located, but how many could survive before more help arrived was anyone's guess. As he pulled out from a low pass over the area, he noticed two of the ship's lifeboats drifting some 2 miles away from the main wreck zone. He flew immediately towards the boats and, doing a quick calculation on his fuel reserve and

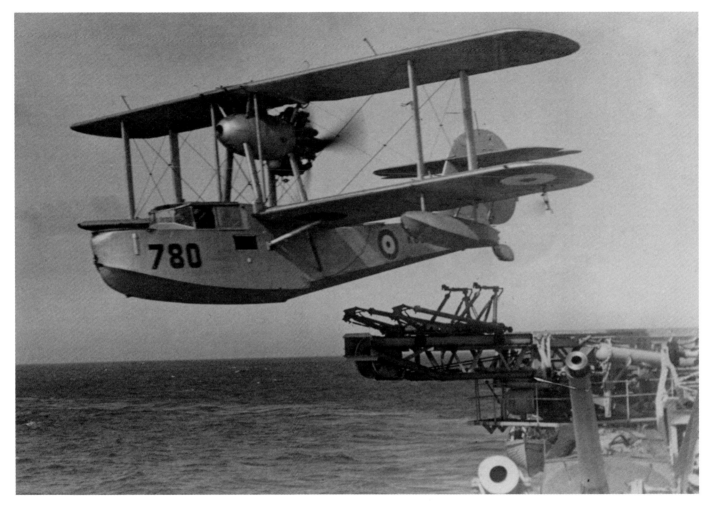

Supermarine Walrus K8341 of No. 718 Sqd, being launched from HMS *Exeter* using a catapult trolley. (FAA Museum)

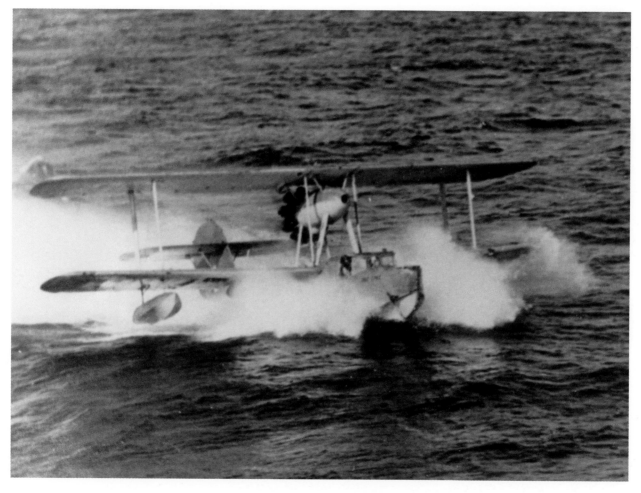

Supermarine Walrus *Just Jake* taxis back alongside HMS *Suffolk*, demonstrating that even in fairly mild sea conditions the aircraft is at risk of becoming waterlogged. (FAA Museum)

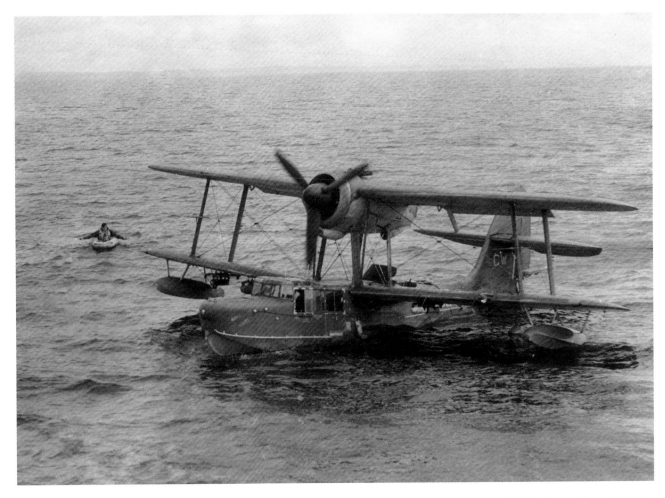

Supermarine Sea Otter *ASR II* of Culdrose Station Flight demonstrating a typical rescue sequence. Ideally it begins by positioning the aircraft on the downwind side of the stranded pilot. (FAA Museum)

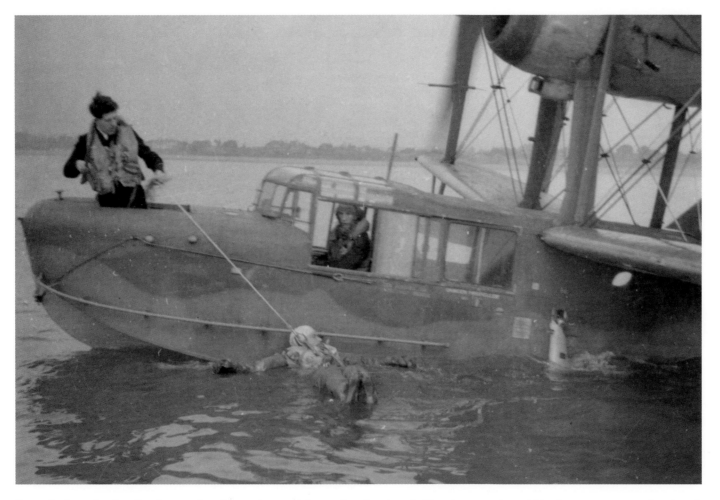

From the front hatch, a line is passed to the survivor and fastened to the aircraft. Note how easy it could be for water to enter the aircraft through the cockpit and forward hatch if sea conditions were rough. (FAA Museum)

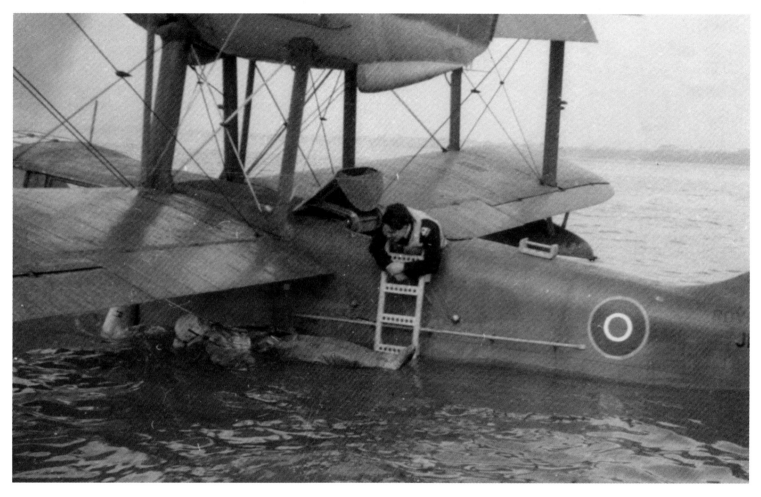

As the aircraft taxis forward, the secured survivor drifts under the wing and alongside the rear hatch to enable easier access or assistance into the aircraft. (FAA Museum)

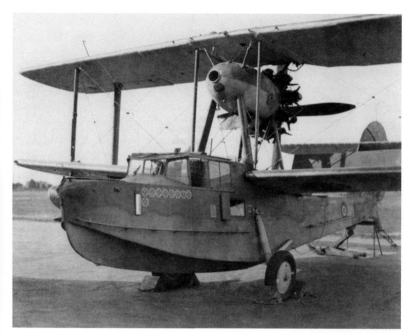

Right: Lifebelts painted as a tally on the nose of the aircraft, with the number of survivors attributed to each rescue mission. (FAA Museum)

Left: Walrus P5658 entered service as an RAF aircraft but was later transferred to the Royal Navy. (FAA Museum).

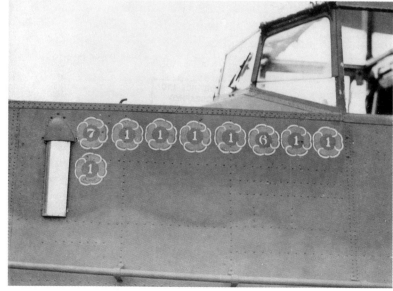

return time, decided he may just have enough fuel to land and perhaps tow the boats back to the stricken men. Approaching closer, he could see that one of the boats had two survivors aboard. The Atlantic swell was considerable and it was not easy to bring the Walrus in to land, but with care he managed to get it down near to the boat with its two bedraggled castaways. Approaching a large wooden lifeboat drifting free is something that any Walrus pilot would be wary of, ever cautious that a collision would almost certainly cause extensive damage to the aircraft's fabric wings, delicate under-wing floats and easily pierced aluminium hull.

As they neared the boat, Cheesman's observer, Petty Officer Knowles, began to ready a rope to throw to the men in the boat to secure a towline. However, the two seamen misunderstood the instructions as they thought that the rope was for them, and so they jumped into the sea and swam for the rope themselves. Once aboard the aircraft they realised their error. One of them was determined to rectify the mistake and aid Lt Cheesman's plan. Back into the water he went, and although it was only a short swim to the lifeboat, he found he was too exhausted to haul himself aboard to secure the line, and again had to be hauled back to the Walrus. Valuable time had now passed. Cheesman abandoned the idea of towing a lifeboat and thought it better to return to the main cluster of survivors before their position was lost. While returning, he rescued two more seamen who had drifted further from the pack, and as he neared the mass of shipwrecked bodies he started to gain a full appreciation of the seriousness of the situation. Manoeuvring carefully amid the wreckage and men in the water, he tried to position the Walrus to enable his observer to pass the aircraft crew's medical kit to a partially submerged lifeboat full of survivors in very poor condition. As he neared the boat the sea swell jarred his aircraft against the boat and badly damaged a wing tip. The damage was severe enough to prevent the Walrus from taking off, and Cheesman and his crew were now stranded along with the shipwrecked survivors. With another Walrus now on hand and circling overhead, thoughts returned to the two lifeboats. Petty Officer Knowles used his Aldis signal lamp to exchange information and get the direction and distance of the nearest of the two boats. With Knowles relaying directions from the forward hatch position, Cheesman set out again to taxi in the direction of the lifeboat and this time bring it back to the struggling survivors.

Having arrived near the boat, there was still the matter of getting a towline secured between boat and aircraft. Cheesman's two crew feared they were not competent enough swimmers and neither of the previously rescued men were in any fit state to assist. With no time to lose Cheesman cut the engine on the Walrus, fastened the line to himself for safety, and dived in, swimming to the boat and securing the towline. To conserve energy he used the line to hand-haul himself back to the aircraft and clambered aboard. After restarting the Walrus engine, they towed the boat back to the other survivors, but this was a tricky manoeuvre with the towline and boat tugging and snatching at the aircraft, making steering difficult and dangerous. Back among the survivors, the boat slowly began to fill with bedraggled, badly sunburned, shocked and traumatised men. As more men made it into the boat, so it became possible for those on board to now manoeuvre the craft without the aid of the Walrus, and so it cast from the aircraft and manoeuvred through the debris field picking up as many more survivors as possible.

The Walrus that had circled overhead a short while before returned and dropped emergency supplies to aid the stranded group; at approximately 1400 hours, some seven hours after Lt Cheesman had arrived on the scene, two trawlers from Freetown harbour were sighted heading to the rescue.

Lt Cheesman's Walrus was put in tow behind one of the trawlers and, very awkwardly and precariously, dragged and buffeted back to Freetown. By dawn the ramshackle convoy had made it to the safety of the harbour; the whole episode had now taken some twenty-four hours, but dozens of men had been saved from certain death amid the treacherous waters of the Southern Atlantic.

Many search and rescue missions had been attempted and accomplished using aircraft during the 1930s and early 1940s, by any squadrons equipped with float planes and seaplanes (notably Nos 700 and 701 Naval Air Squadrons), as SAR duties became an ever more necessary support service within the Fleet Air Arm.

In November 1944, No. 1700 Naval Air Squadron formed at Lee-on-Solent, Hampshire. This squadron's main role was that of amphibious bomber reconnaissance, completing mine-sweeping tasks using Supermarine Walrus aircraft. However, SAR tasks were now very much a part of their duties, with the squadron badge clearly indicating this role. The badge depicted an anchor over waves, with two arms reaching from the water and clutching the anchor for safety. The Latin inscribed moto reading *Ex Mari Messis:* 'Our Harvest is From the Sea'.

Throughout the Second World War, many new ideas and innovations for improved rescue techniques were tried. One of the more unusual was that of a lifeboat being dropped by parachute from beneath an aircraft.

These air-dropped lifeboats were the invention of British boat builder and designer Uffa Fox, and were employed by both RAF and Royal Navy aircraft with varying degrees of success. Using a fast, long-range aircraft to search of a missing aircrew would be a distinct advantage over the Walrus if it were then possible to deliver the stranded crew a useful-sized lifeboat.

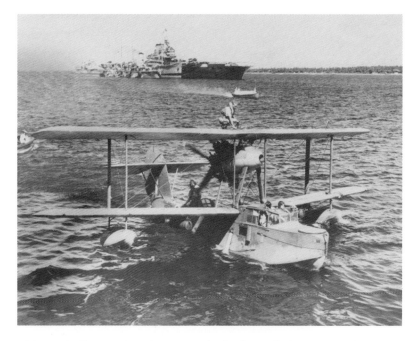

Walrus of No. 710 Squadron taxis back alongside her parent ship HMS *Albatross* in Freetown harbour, 1940. The crewman on the top wing is waiting to attach the crane hook to the lifting point to enable the aircraft to be hoisted back onto the mother ship. (FAA Museum)

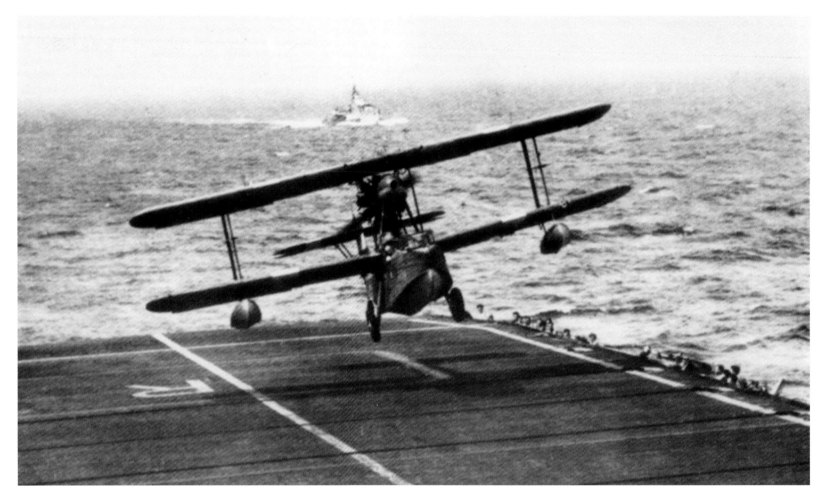

Battling against high winds, Lt F. Lawrence arrives safely back onto the deck of HMS *Ameer* in the ship's Walrus aircraft, having just rescued a downed No. 896 Squadron Hellcat pilot from hostile Japanese waters, July 1945. (FAA Museum)

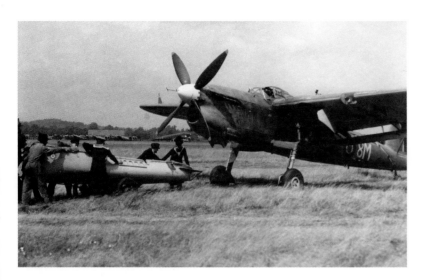

Ground crews at RNAS Easthaven manhandle an Uffa-Fox lifeboat into position on the underside of a Fairey Barracuda II. (FAA Museum)

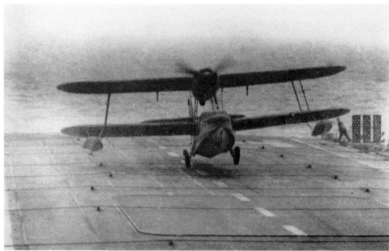

Sea Otter *Neptune's Daughter*, piloted by Lt Cdr Cane, lands back onto *HMS Triumph* during the Korean War. (FAA Museum).

The boat, complete with food and survival equipment, would descend by parachute and was designed to be self-righting when on the water. The Royal Navy trialled the idea using Fairey Barracuda aircraft, attaching the boat to the underside of the fuselage on modified torpedo attachment points. The concept was interesting, but had its limitations. Weight was an issue, and there were also problems with accurately dropping the boat close enough to a stranded crew for them to reach it, but not so close as to endanger them from its descent onto the water. A boat that is maybe as near as 50–60 metres might as well be 50 miles away if it is drifting out of reach or they are injured, too cold, or too tired to be able to reach it.

Getting in as close as was possible with seaplanes still afforded the best chances of survival and rescue for stranded airmen, provided sea conditions allowed a safe landing. Fixed-wing aircraft were still of great value to fly swiftly to extended range and locate someone in peril or guide a vessel to their assistance, but were otherwise beginning to reach the end of their capabilities for rescue tasks. It would take the arrival of the helicopter to make significant changes in all aspects of supporting the Navy, and in search and rescue in particular.

Fairey Barracuda with an Uffa Fox lifeboat attached to the aircraft where a torpedo would normally be carried. (FAA Museum)

One rescue carried by out by Royal Navy pilot Lt Cane and his observer G. O'Nion in July 1950 during the Korean War fittingly brings the era of the Walrus and Otter to a close as fixed-wing SAR began to give way to the age of the helicopter rescue.

American pilot Lt Boyd Muncie had been shot down in his F-4U Corsair fighter plane after a sortie over North Korea, and was now floating in icy cold and extremely hostile enemy waters. Lt Muncie's wingman stayed circling overhead in his own Corsair, acting as a marker while a Sea Otter, JM960, was sent immediately from the British aircraft carrier HMS *Triumph* to attempt a rescue. In atrocious and marginal conditions, the two man team managed to battle through bad weather and land their Sea Otter in rough seas and severe gusting winds to perform the rescue. The sea was so rough that Lt Cane (now flying very low) was unable to perform a normal landing because of the height and severity of the waves. Instead, he had to effectively bring his aircraft all but to a halt in flight and drop it into a trough in the waves amid the heavy swell. Taking off was similarly difficult, and to get airborne Lt Cane had to plough through the heaving waves until he had just enough forward speed to almost bounce the little aircraft off the waves and back into the air. A short time later they arrived safely back on HMS *Triumph* with Lt Muncie safe, amazed, but uninjured. As well as being a significant joint services Anglo-American combat rescue, it was also the last rescue performed by a Sea Otter. The Sea Otter was retired from service in early 1952, bringing to a close many years of Royal Navy fixed-wing amphibian duties.

3

BIRTH OF HELICOPTER RESCUE

Often considered to be an invention of the 1950s, the helicopter was more advanced during the Second World War than many people realise.

In November 1943, with the war raging on all fronts and some seven months before the D-Day landings, Britain and America were conducting joint service flight trials (US Coast Guard Unit, Royal Navy and Royal Air Force) with the new American Sikorsky design, the R-4 helicopter. The trials included extensive experiments at various American air bases, in Brooklyn Harbour (using float equipped R-4s) and from a small deck on the converted cargo vessel the SS *Daghestan*. The outcome was so successful that Royal Navy and RAF training schools were equipped with R-4s during 1944 and by May 1945 two Hoverfly helicopters (as they were now known) were attached to No. 771 Naval Air Squadron.

On 7 May 1947, helicopter duties and evaluation fell under the control of the newly reformed No. 705 Naval Air Squadron. No. 705 NAS became responsible for all Fleet Air Arm helicopter pilot training, special trials and SAR training and became the first all-helicopter equipped squadron of the Royal Navy. The age of the helicopter had truly arrived.

Test Pilot Captain Eric Brown RN CBE DSC AFC recalls that as a test pilot attached to Aerodynamics Flight, RAE Farnborough, he was among the very few pilots to test-fly the Hoverfly helicopter when it first arrived in Britain. Although it was tricky to master at first, he could immediately see the potential that the helicopter could offer:

There was no doubt in my mind that the helicopter was a gift from Heaven for search and rescue work, and effective plane guard duties on carriers was now going to be possible. The helicopter was an immense step forward and was going to transform Carrier [aircraft carrier] safety.

The task of 'plane guard duty' is to provide a rapid response rescue crew to assist, should an aircraft taking off or landing on an aircraft carrier crash into the sea as the result of an accident. The crashed pilot's life would depend almost entirely on the

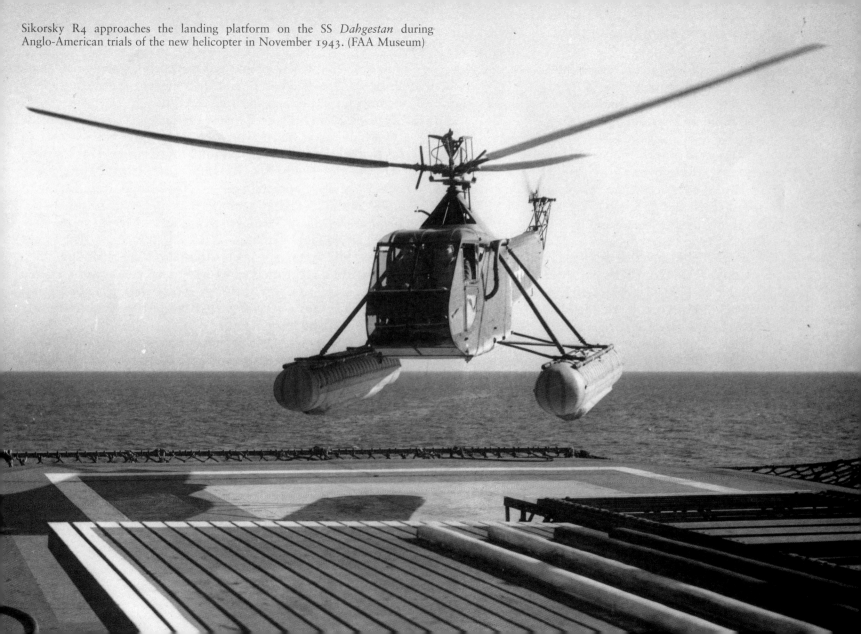

Sikorsky R4 approaches the landing platform on the SS *Dahgestan* during Anglo-American trials of the new helicopter in November 1943. (FAA Museum)

speed at which the plane guard rescue crew could reach him. If the pilot were injured or trapped inside of his aircraft, then there would be less than minutes to free him and rescue him. Prior to 1950, pilots could only rely on a plane guard being provided by a crew of twelve men in a large wooden rowing boat (known as a whaler) waiting to launch from a destroyer or similar small ship shadowing a little to the rear and off to the left of the aircraft carrier. Should an accident occur, the destroyer would have to adjust speed and direction towards the crash site, lower the whaler as swiftly as possible and then the boat crew would have to row like fury the last distance and try to rescue the pilot.

Having a helicopter hovering near the carrier during flying stations, with a fully trained rescue diver on board, would mean that in the event of an aircraft crashing into the sea, the helicopter could swoop in seconds and deliver the rescue diver right onto the target and then remain on station in the hover ready to recover both airman and diver back to safety. This huge improvement in response time and safety would save many more airmen's lives, and would be significantly more cost effective than having another small ship shadow a carrier for this temporary and intermittent task.

During the early years of naval aviation, one incident that provided a very stark demonstration for such a need occurred in August 1917 when Sqd Cdr E. H. Dunning was performing the very first deck landings onto a moving ship. His first two attempts were successful, but tragically on his third attempt his Sopwith aircraft veered over the side of HMS *Furious* and plunged into the sea. A flotation bag in the tail of the aircraft prevented it from sinking completely, but Dunning had been knocked out with the impact of the crash. By the time HMS *Furious* had

slowed, steered a new course and launched a rescue boat, some twenty minutes had passed and Dunning had drowned, trapped unconscious in the cockpit of his aircraft.

A plane guard helicopter waiting in the hover could have made a vital difference, but it would be some thirty years before an effective helicopter had been invented and developed for such use.

During the 1940s, the R-4 Hoverfly was still very much undergoing development and evaluation and was too small to effectively operate as a full SAR or plane guard helicopter. However, extensive low-level flying and hovering trials were being carried out, exploring different techniques that might prove useful for rescuing people from different situations.

These trials and experiments were a necessary and valuable part of getting to know this new rotary-wing technology and integrating it into a service (and a world) that had previously only known fixed-wing aircraft.

By the mid- to late 1940s, the Sikorsky Company was leading the world in helicopter design and manufacture, and the successor to their R-4 design, the X-5, had already been test flown by 1946. The X-5 quickly developed into the Sikorsky H-5 as a production helicopter, ultimately becoming the Sikorsky S-51. In 1947 Westland Aircraft Ltd, England, acquired the build rights to manufacture the S-51 for the British market, naming it the Dragonfly. This contract marked the start of a thirty-year production run of Sikorsky designs produced under licence by the Westland Company.

The Dragonfly was an instant success and a significant development over the Hoverfly, and by 1949 Dragonfly helicopters operated by No. 194 Squadron RAF were being used for casevac (casualty evacuation) in Malaya.

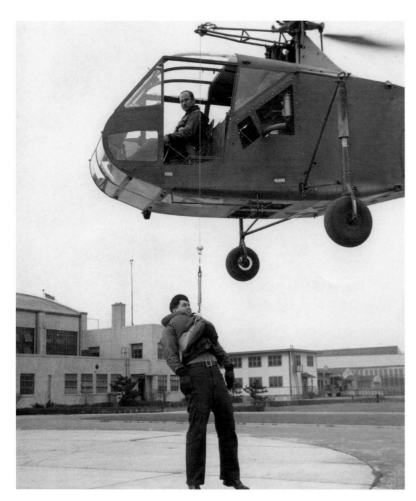

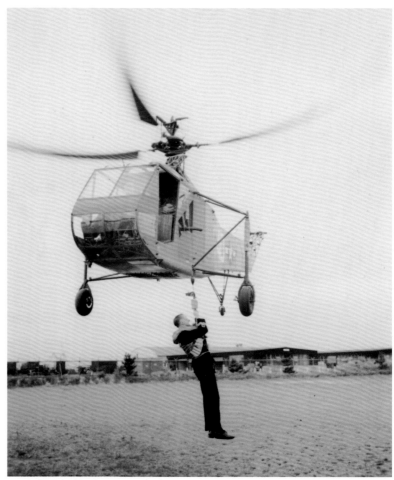

Lt Cdr Peat, RNVR, being winched by a US Navy Sikorsky R4 during a demonstration for the United States Coast Guard Service, 1944. (FAA Museum)

US Navy Sikorsky R4 demonstrating a very low-level winching operation, 1944. (FAA Museum)

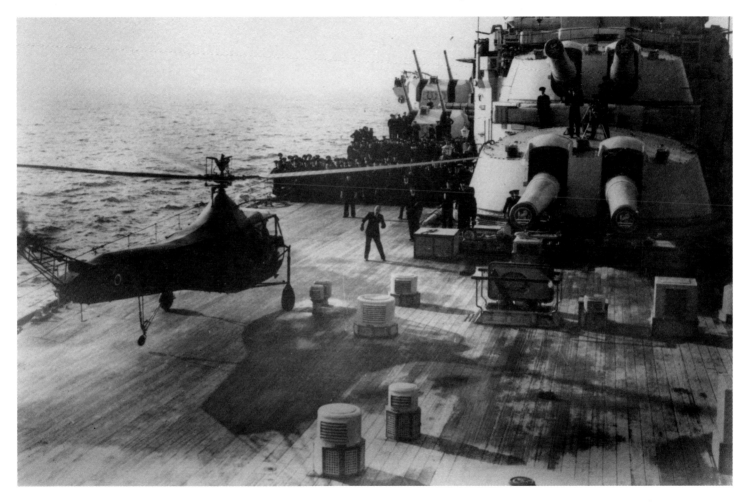

1 February 1947 and Lt K. Reed makes the first helicopter landing onto a Royal Navy ship underway at sea (HMS *Vanguard*). There is no proper landing platform, only a cleared deck space precariously close to the ship's guns. (FAA Museum)

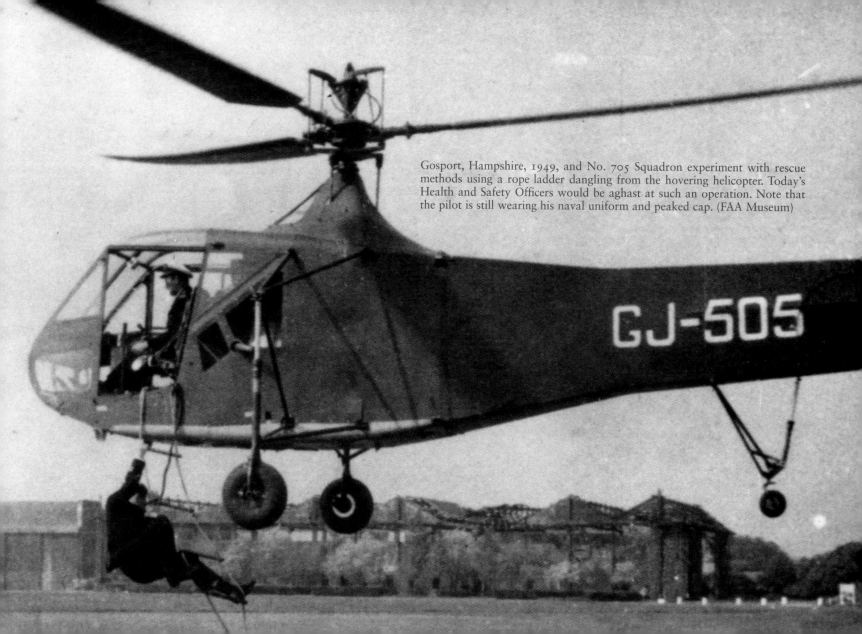

Gosport, Hampshire, 1949, and No. 705 Squadron experiment with rescue methods using a rope ladder dangling from the hovering helicopter. Today's Health and Safety Officers would be aghast at such an operation. Note that the pilot is still wearing his naval uniform and peaked cap. (FAA Museum)

The Dragonfly was considerably larger than the Hoverfly, with an increase in engine power from 200 hp to 550 hp. This increase in size and power enabled the Dragonfly to be used immediately for effective plane guard duties and, with a range of 300 miles, could now perform effective SAR tasks.

However, much of that increased engine power was absorbed by lifting the weight of the larger airframe, larger fuel tank, extra equipment (including a rescue winch), a co-pilot/winch operator and, of course, a rescued (often soaking wet) person, so there were still limitations. As mentioned earlier, time spent hovering uses considerably more fuel than in cruising flight, as does flying in high winds or difficult conditions, any of which the pilot may experience during an SAR mission. The reference to the rescued person being soaking wet is also quite significant. In certain conditions, where the helicopter may be struggling to maintain lift or is on the edge of its capability, a rescued person wearing a waterlogged sheepskin flying jacket and clothes would noticeably affect the lifting capacity of the helicopter. Helicopter technology was developing at an enormous rate, but it was also highlighting how important engine power and overall aircraft weight was to sustained and useful performance. This would be the main area of concern and development for all helicopter manufacturers from 1950 onwards.

Reference has already been made to the Korean War and the valuable work performed by the Sea Otter. However, the Korean War was to be the proving ground for the helicopter as a battlefield tool. American forces used the H-5 (S-51) extensively from the outset of this conflict for communications, transporting vital supplies, casualty evacuation and SAR. As useful as fixed-wing aircraft were at transporting casualties to medical units or field hospitals, there was often a critical delay in getting the injured person to a safe landing strip and onto an aircraft. Helicopter pilots would still have to negotiate uncertain and often hostile landing zones, and the lifting capacity was still limited, but being able to access the battlefield directly and exit with your casualty back to a field hospital at speeds of up to 100 mph significantly reduced the mortality rate of downed pilots or troops with serious injuries.

On 11 October 1950, a Sikorsky H-5 helicopter piloted by 1st Lt David C. McDaniel (US 3rd Air Rescue Service) picked up

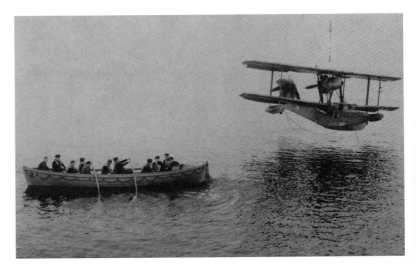

Walrus crew being transported between an aircraft and ship using a ship's life boat, or 'Whaler' as they were known. Before helicopters, this would have been the only means of attending a crashed aircraft to hopefully rescue the pilot. (FAA Museum)

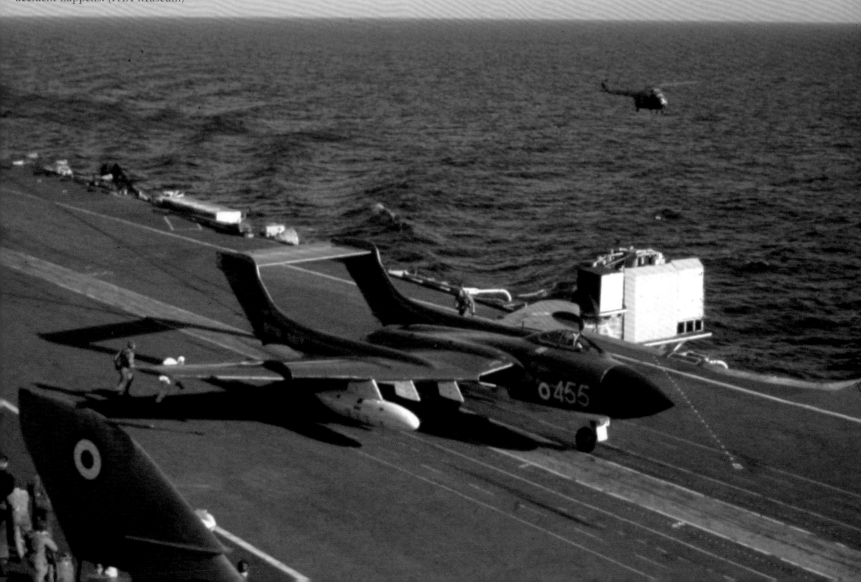

A Sea Vixen makes a safe landing onto HMS *Ark Royal* while the plane guard helicopter hovers on station and ready to respond at a moment's notice if an accident happens. (FAA Museum)

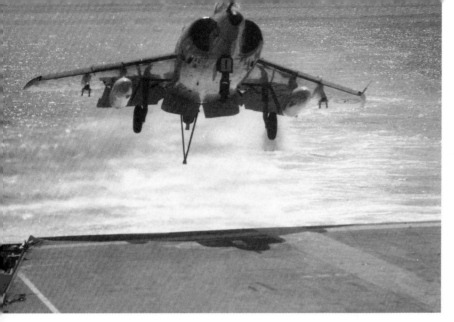

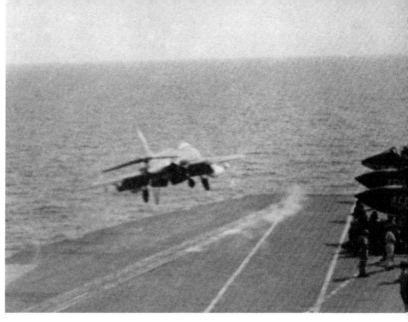

Top left: When it all goes wrong: a Supermarine Scimitar comes in to land on HMS *Centaur*.

Top right and bottom left: It misses the last arrestor wire and plunges over the side of the flight deck and into the sea. (FAA Museum)

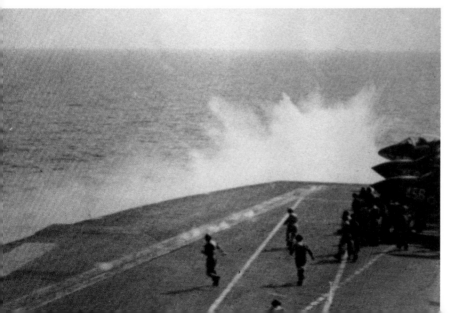

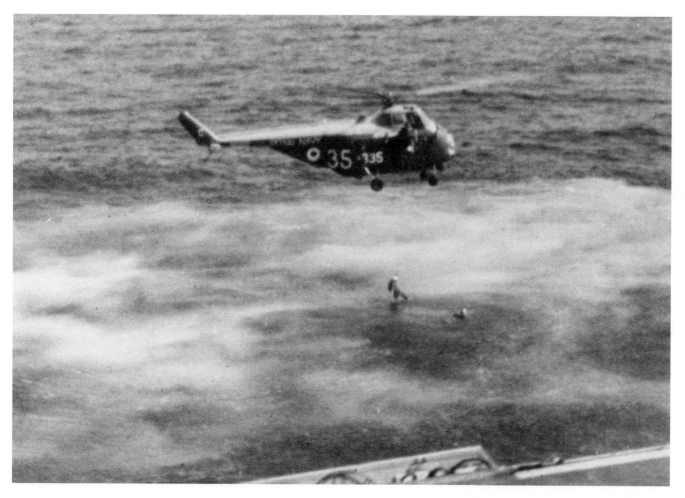

Saved! The plane guard helicopter swoops to the aid of the crashed aircraft in seconds. The aircraft has barely submerged as the winchman is lowered to rescue the pilot. (FAA Museum)

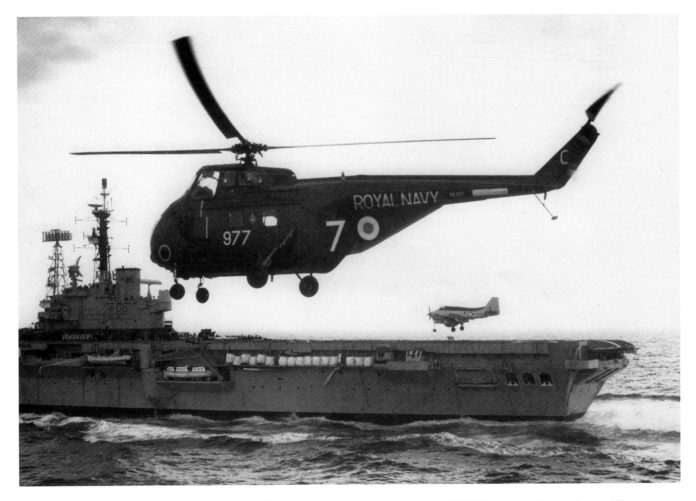

The age of the plane guard helicopter. Whirlwind XK912 in position off the port side of *HMS Centaur* as Fairey Gannet XL502 comes in on finals. (FAA Museum)

British Navy pilot Lt Stanley Leonard when he was shot down on a raid over North Korea. Four Sea Fury aircraft from No. 807 Naval Air Squadron had been attacking North Korean positions when Leonard's aircraft was hit by ground fire. Leonard was able to make a forced landing in a paddy field, but the aircraft broke up on impact, leaving him seriously injured and trapped in the wreckage. Stuck behind enemy lines, his only chance of survival now would be a helicopter rescue. The remaining Sea Furies radioed for assistance and stayed overhead to mark the spot and provide what air-to-ground cover they could, while Lt McDaniel flew low and fast from Kimpo airfield to the crash site in his H-5 helicopter, a journey that took about one hour.

McDaniel was able to land his helicopter within 150 yards of the injured airman, allowing para-doctor Captain John C. Shumate (McDaniel's crew man) to race to his aid. Under enemy fire, Shumate managed to drag, carry and bundle the injured pilot out of the crashed Sea Fury, across the paddy field and into the helicopter. Leonard was bleeding badly and Shumate began administering blood plasma to the wounded man as the helicopter took off. This was the first time a blood plasma transfusion had been performed in flight in a helicopter. Such rescues were to be repeated time and again, and by the end of the conflict in 1953 helicopters had been responsible for recovering over 7,000 seriously injured soldiers and nearly 1,000 men trapped behind enemy lines.

1953 would be a significant year for the helicopter; while it was demonstrating its worth as a battlefield support vehicle in Korea, it was also being used for humanitarian aid much closer to home. In January and February 1953, a combination of bad weather and extremely high tides caused extensive flooding in the coastal regions of eastern England and the Netherlands, leaving hundreds of people stranded and homeless. Access was difficult by boat and impossible by roads, as most were impassable or had been swept away. The most useful fast response vehicle available was the helicopter, and on 31 January 1953 the Royal Navy dispatched Dragonfly HR1 and HR3 helicopters of No. 705 NAS to respond to the urgent need for assistance. The helicopter was again to prove invaluable for flying over flooded areas and for spotting stranded

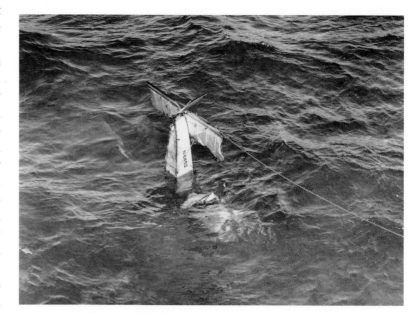

The tail of Squadron Commander E. H. Dunning's Sopwith Pup protrudes from the water after his tragic accident. Today's plane guard helicopters help to prevent such scenarios turning into tragic fatalities. (FAA Museum)

people, with many being rescued from the roof tops of buildings that were all but submerged. Food and urgent medical supplies could be flown in, or dropped onto dry areas for collection, and stranded people and casualties air lifted out. Over 840 people were rescued by helicopter during the flood crisis, sixty-four of these being rooftop rescues. During this frantic series of ferry flights and rescue sorties, one pilot rescued 111 flood victims during one seven-hour period of flying, with another managing 102. Considering that the Dragonfly had a typical one hour maximum flying time between re-fuelling, and could rescue only one or at the most two people at a time, these were phenomenal achievements by any measure. At the end of the crisis the Commanding Officer of No. 705 NAS, Lt Cdr Spedding, and his accompanying crewman, Sydney Craig, were awarded an MBE and BEM respectively in recognition of their efforts. All of No. 705 NAS crews worked to the maximum during this crisis and an extract from Lt Ronald Crayton's flying log book clearly demonstrates how busy, varied and dangerous their flying was during this time. Flying rescue sorties and ferrying doctors, equipment and food supplies were the daily routine. However, as the log book shows on 8 February, helicopter flying in adverse conditions could turn from difficult to disastrous in seconds. The entry describes a landing onto the bank of a dyke, with limited space and in icy conditions at Achthuizen in the southern Netherlands: 'ACHTHUIZEN. A/C [aircraft] skidded on ice on dyke and crashed into the sea. Both passengers unhurt. Paddled ashore in A/C dinghy'. The passengers referred to were two Dutch armed forces personnel and miraculously all escaped without injury.

'Search and Rescue' had now been a recognised element of many squadrons' duties since the end of the First World War, but the arrival of the helicopter and its use in Korea and the floods of 1953 seems to be the defining moment when 'search and rescue' became a household phrase, synonymous with the helicopter and its place in modern aviation. The Royal Navy and the RAF, along with many other nations' military and civilian operators, would all now focus on the helicopter to develop this role.

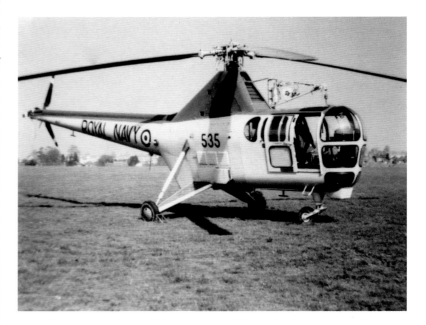

Rare colour image of a Westland Dragonfly helicopter. Dragonflys entered service with an all-over silver colour scheme. Later schemes adopted were either sky lower surface and dark-sea-grey upper surface (like this HR-3) or all-over glossy sea-blue. (FAA Museum)

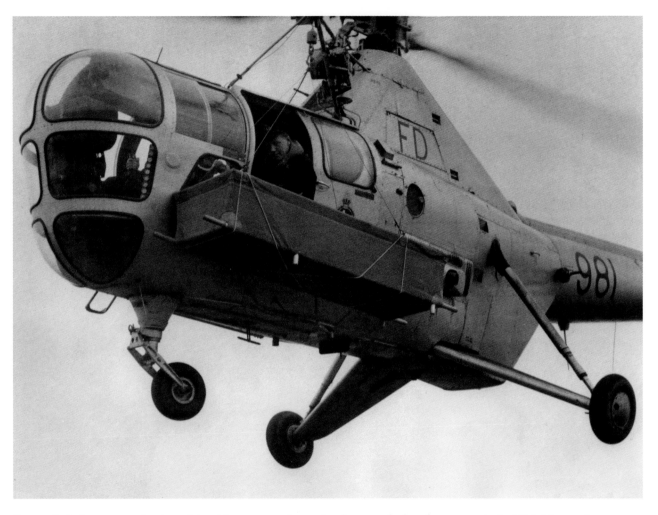

Dragonfly helicopter conducting trials with an external stretcher box attached to the rescue winch. (FAA Museum)

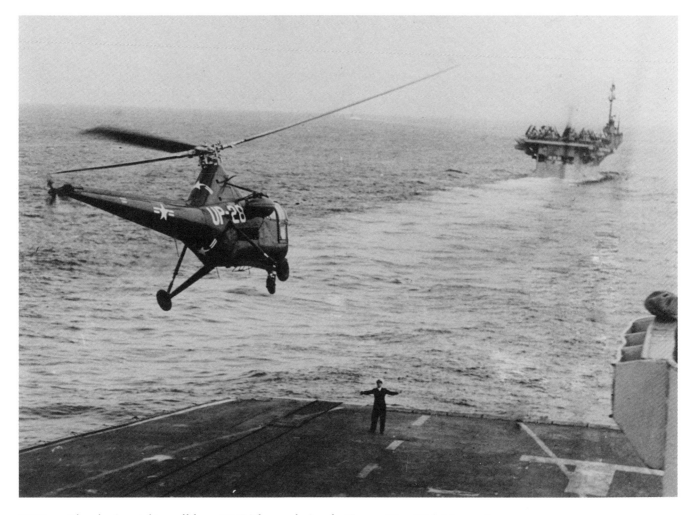

US Navy Sikorsky S-51 taking off from HMS *Theseus* during the Korean War. (FAA Museum)

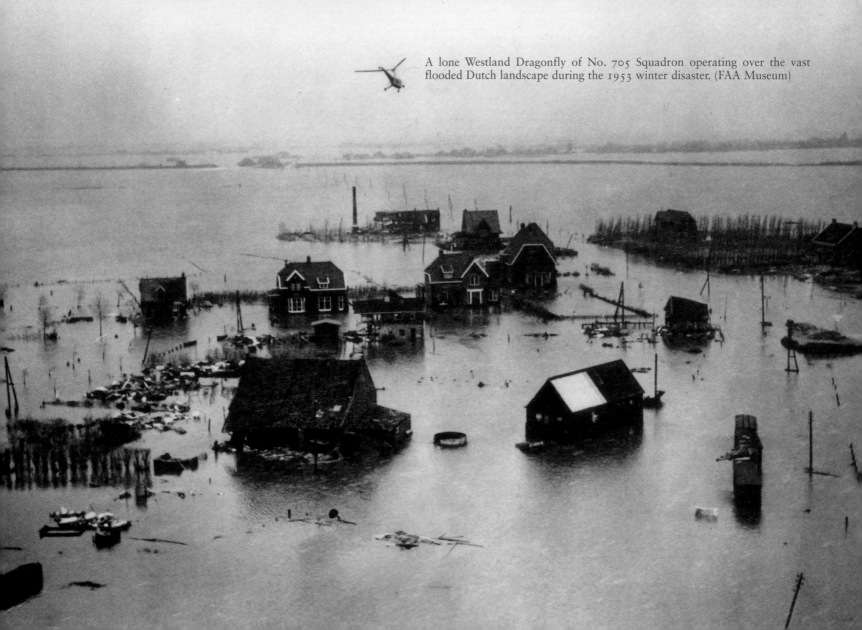

A lone Westland Dragonfly of No. 705 Squadron operating over the vast flooded Dutch landscape during the 1953 winter disaster. (FAA Museum)

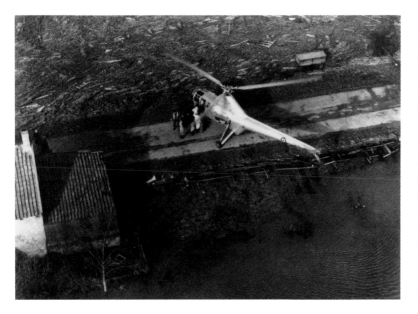

Landing crossways, on a small raised track way amid the floods, a No. 705 Squadron Dragonfly HR1 picks up stranded Dutch civilians during the 1953 floods. (FAA Museum)

The Royal Navy soon equipped seven of its UK air stations with search and rescue (SAR) helicopters. With trained SAR crews based in the North West (Cumbria), Wales, Northern Ireland, East Scotland, Sussex, Hampshire and Cornwall, they could provide emergency response over the length and breadth of Britain, and a considerable distance out to sea.

The Dragonfly set a new benchmark for all helicopter designs and each successive new Sikorsky design would bring massive improvements in speed, range and lifting capabilities. The helicopter was now as much a part of military and civilian flying as any other aircraft type that had gone before.

Countless hundreds of helicopter SAR and casevac missions have been achieved since the introduction of the Dragonfly and it would be impossible to list them all. Indeed some conflicts, such as the Malayan Emergency 1948–1960, would see no fewer than three new helicopter designs (Westland Dragonfly, Whirlwind and Wessex) used during this extended twelve-year period of unrest. The following chapters are a selection of instances that help to describe the variety and diversity of calls that Royal Navy pilots have been asked to respond to.

4

WESTLAND DRAGONFLY

Test pilot Captain Eric Brown experienced first-hand the benefits that a helicopter could bring to those quite literally in peril on the sea. While he was stationed at Brawdy in west Wales during the winter of 1955, his squadron was called to the assistance of a stricken Greek cargo vessel approximately 15 miles off shore. Captain Brown recalls:

We had a call one afternoon that a Greek container ship was in trouble and breaking up about 15 miles off shore. The weather was absolutely terrible, so bad that we had to start the helicopters up in the hangar and taxi them out, it was too rough to start them up outside.

We took off and headed out towards the ship, I was in the lead helicopter. On the way we were told that the ship had all but broken in two, so I said that I would take the forward end and directed the second helicopter to concentrate on the rear section.

In those days we had made water proof pouches with instructions showing someone how to attach themselves to the rescue line. I sent mine down attached to the hook, so they could look at the pictures and see how to put the harness over their head and shoulders. To my alarm, the first man took the pouch off the hook and then attached the hook to the guard rail while he studied the picture. I was now attached to a sinking ship! I could have cut the cable from my end, but of course did not want to as I would not have been able to rescue anyone.

Somehow I managed to signal to unhook me from the ship and to put the harness on, which the first man did eventually do. I had flown out without an aircrewman for the first flight to save weight and hoping I would be able to pick up two survivors. However, operating the winch and controlling the aircraft, was to prove too difficult and I was only able to rescue one at a time. On the next run out we took an aircrew winch operator in each helicopter, which added more weight in the extreme conditions and still limited us to picking up one person at a time, but did mean we were each able to pick up survivors more quickly.

There were seven men on my end of the ship. However, we were only 15 miles offshore, so we went back and forth as swiftly as we could until all were rescued, we managed to get them all off safely, but we were exhausted by the time we had finished, flying the Dragonfly in extreme weather conditions and accurately enough to lift men from the deck of a sinking ship takes a great deal of concentration and effort.

In another incident, he recalls carrying out the recovery of a seriously ill crewman from a submarine in the Irish Sea, again using the Dragonfly helicopter to perform the task:

It was while I was on HMS *Illustrious*, we were in the Irish Sea and got a signal that one of the crew of the submarine *Tally-Ho* was very ill with peritonitis and needed very urgent treatment. I flew out from the ship in the Dragonfly and picked the poor chap up. We had to do the pick up with the sub still moving into wind, so we could use the advantage of flying into wind for extra lift. We had to do this to cope with the extra weight of man and stretcher. I had to take a crewman with me to manoeuvre the stretcher and patient, and with this extra weight we were just about up to lift capacity. I had to get down to about 30 feet above the deck of the submarine and aft of the conning tower, and then stay in the hover, but moving forwards with the sub. There was a lot of turbulence and disturbed air around the tower, so I had to be aware of this during what was a tricky operation. We managed to hoist the stretcher up, but of course the Dragonfly fuselage is not that wide, and so the crewman

had to get the stretcher in as best he could, and we headed off to Belfast Hospital with a part of the stretcher sticking out of the doorway.

The experience from the other end of the rescue line can be equally dramatic and fraught with its own problems and dangers. Lt Graham Foster recalls that when he was a pilot, flying Hawker Sea Fury aircraft during the 1950s, he had to

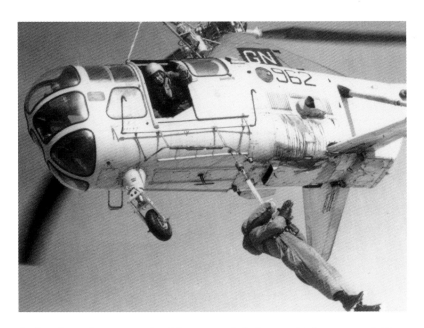

A view from the rescue wire. Many stranded airmen, ship's crew or civilians have been very relieved to see a Dragonfly looming overhead and providing what may have been their only chance of survival. (FAA Museum).

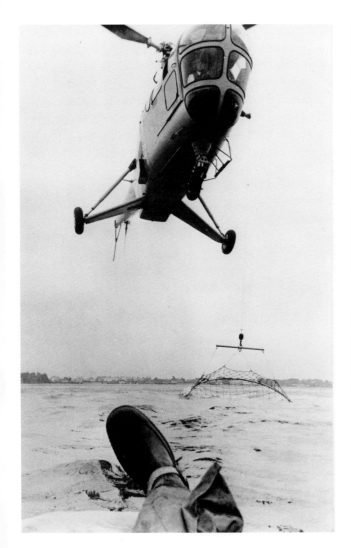

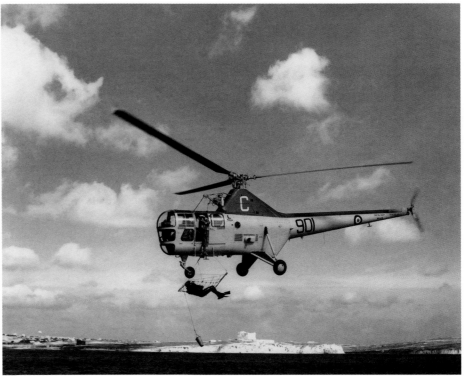

Above: Dragonfly WG671 from HMS *Centaur*, practicing picking up a Royal Navy diver using a Sproule net. (FAA Museum)

Left: 'Sproule net' trials. Inching forward in a low hover, the Dragonfly trawls its Sproule net through the water, ready to scoop a stranded airman to safety. (FAA Museum)

make two 'ditchings' (forced landings in the sea), interestingly within only a few days of each other. He witnessed first-hand the transition from rescue by boat to rescue by helicopter.

He recalls,

On the 20th October some twelve days after my first ditching and rescue by boat, I was again airborne from HMS *Theseus* doing target practice firing off the stern of the ship. At the end of the training session I began to experience engine trouble again, and again observed failing oil pressure.

The ship instructed me to head for the airfield at Hal-Far on Malta, which was about twenty minutes flying time away, so I set off towards Malta but after a short time was losing oil rapidly and the engine was close to stopping. I prepared myself to ditch again. Fortunately the sea was flat calm and the Fury touched down and skated over the surface to a standstill. I scrambled out and got into my dinghy and as the aircraft sank beneath me I floated and waited to be picked up. A Short Sturgeon aircraft from Hal-Far arrived and circled overhead, so I knew I had been located. Then a helicopter appeared in the distance coming from Hal-Far and heading my way and I launched my Very pistol red flares as an additional marker.

We were all familiar with helicopters in service by this time and I suspected that it may be a helicopter that came to pick me up, although it was the first time I would have experienced it.

Most people just take for granted that a helicopter arrives and picks you up, but in those early days of helicopter rescues there was a lot that could go wrong.

The air temperature was very hot that day, there was absolutely no wind and the surface of the water was like glass. You would think that was perfect, but in fact these were very difficult conditions for the Dragonfly to operate in. As the helicopter came in close and tried to hover, the downdraft from the rotors blew me in my dinghy across the calm surface and away from the helicopter. This happened a few times until I realised that I was going to have to get into the water and away from the dinghy to allow the helicopter to position itself over me. The winch-man sent down the line and harness and I slipped it over my head and under my arms. However, the Dragonfly was having great trouble trying to get enough engine power in the very hot and still air to perform an accurate and steady hover. Added to that the lifting capacity of the helicopter with pilot (he was a big man as I recall) his winch-man and the added weight of me in the water was actually too much for the helicopter to lift. As the winch man attempted to raise me I remember hearing the engine making some very odd straining noises as the weight of me being drawn from the water loaded the helicopter further, and rather than me going up, the helicopter was actually being winched down towards the sea. Without some head wind and in such hot still air, I was just too much for the helicopter to lift out from the water, soaking wet, it really was that marginal. The winch-man let out the line again and signalled that they would have to make a transition into forward flight and use the forward motion to generate more lift and pull me clear of the water. I sort of understood what he was signalling to me, but had no time to think much about it, and they had little time to reiterate their signal and intention. The next thing I knew the nose of the helicopter dipped, the engine roared, and suddenly I was being towed through the water, gaining speed and being sloshed and buffeted around. It seemed like a great distance, but probably was not far, but it was jolly uncomfortable. Finally the helicopter had generated enough forward speed to increase its lift and I was at last out of the water, dangling in mid air and now flying at about sixty to seventy miles per hour.

As the helicopter levelled out to cruise, I was winched up to the doorway and the winch-man twirled me around on the hook and sat me on the ledge with my legs hanging out through the door. There was nowhere to sit inside really, I just sat half out of the door for the flight back to the ship. On the way back to the ship the winch-man leaned across and shouted into my ear, 'For a minute I thought we were coming in to join you!' Yes early helicopter rescues were quite precarious and although many lives were saved by the speed and effectiveness of the helicopter it was not always as easy as you might think.

Constantly trying to improve methods and techniques of rescue was an ongoing challenge for all helicopter squadrons and for No. 705 NAS in particular. One innovative member of the squadron, Lt Cdr John Sproule, was very aware of the problem that Lt Foster had experienced and the often limited lift capacity of the Dragonfly. His invention of a scoop-shaped net (known as the Sproule net) could be lowered from a helicopter to literally scoop a person from the water. It was a basic and quirky solution, but worked well. The Sproule net remained in use with the Royal Navy from the 1950s until the early 1970s. Similar devices are still used by some countries for SAR and Special Forces units today.

5

WESTLAND WHIRLWIND

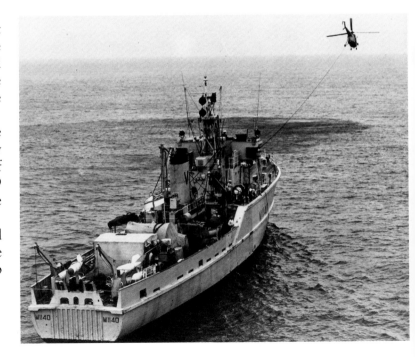

While the Dragonfly was still relatively new in service, the next generation of Sikorsky designs was beginning to roll off the Westland helicopter production line. The Westland Whirlwind was again a licence-built copy of a Sikorsky design, this time the type S-55, and would take helicopter operations into a whole new level of capability and performance.

The Whirlwind anti-submarine helicopter would evolve through a number of mark changes in its lifetime, from a few early Sikorsky types transferred to the Navy, through a series of British built Mk 3, Mk 5, Mk 7 and Mk 9 versions. The Mk 9 would see the transition from a piston engine to a gas turbine engine, another huge technological advance.

The Whirlwind was physically larger than the Dragonfly and was capable of carrying up to four people in addition to the three man crew. The engine horsepower had increased by some 200 hp

Whirlwind XG582 is worked to the limit pulling the Ton-class Minesweeper M1140 in this extreme experiment to evaluate whether a helicopter could pull a stricken ship to safety. (FAA Museum).

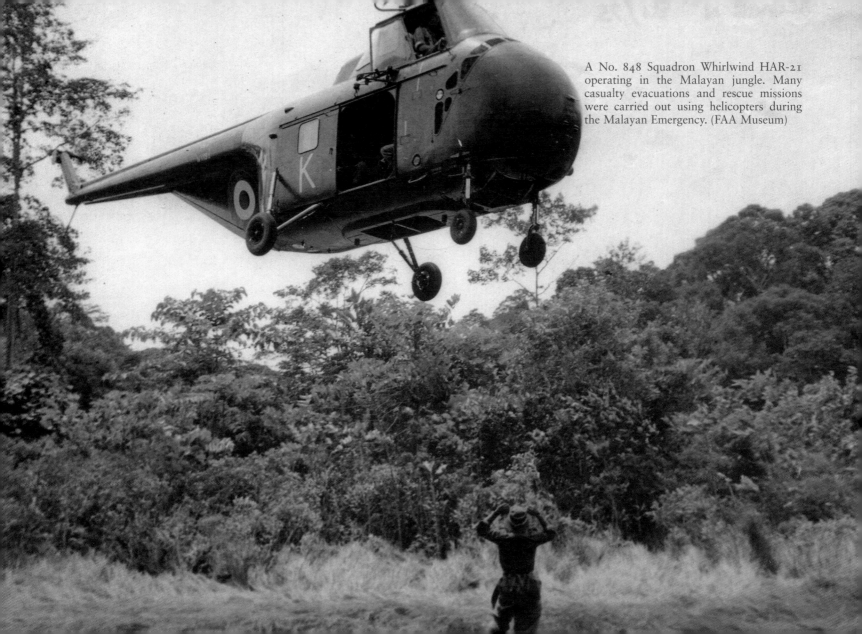

A No. 848 Squadron Whirlwind HAR-21 operating in the Malayan jungle. Many casualty evacuations and rescue missions were carried out using helicopters during the Malayan Emergency. (FAA Museum)

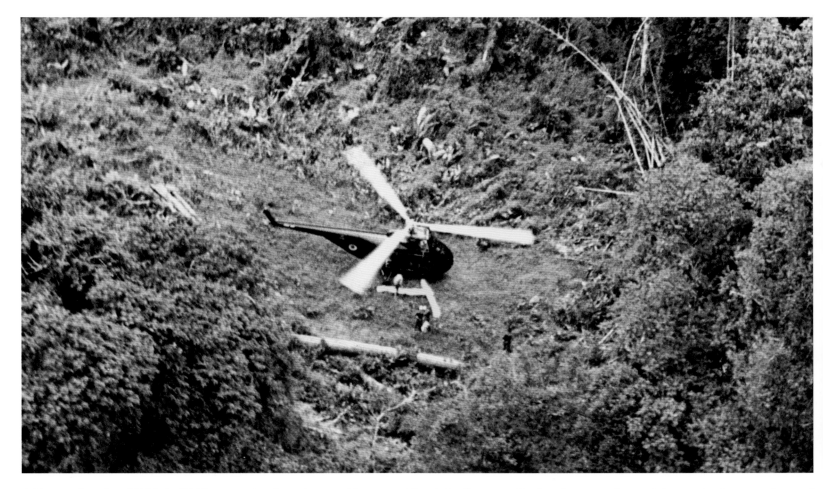

A No. 848 Squadron Whirlwind HAR-21 touches down in a roughly prepared jungle landing zone. Getting close enough to a pick up point for a casualty amid the Malayan jungle was a constant challenge for the pilots and the men on the ground. Yellow 'T' markers identify the centre of the landing zone and indicate the direction of the wind. (FAA Museum)

over the Dragonfly, taking it to around 750 hp. This provided more lift capacity that could be translated directly into increased fuel load and therefore greater range and flight duration, or a lift capacity that could now deal with small under-slung loads (with lower fuel loads).

Helicopter development had reached a new age and although every new design will have its own new shortfalls and limitations, the Whirlwind was a vast improvement over the earlier Dragonfly.

By the mid-1950s helicopters were a permanent element of aircraft carrier operations and were also accompanying many smaller Royal Navy vessels and support ships where a landing pad and hangar space could be configured. One such vessel was HMS *Protector*, a former 1930s net-laying and target-towing ship, converted for patrolling Antarctic waters and assisting with geological survey work. Patrolling these waters had previously been carried out by Royal Navy destroyers without the additional benefit of helicopter support. The advent of HMS *Protector*, and her ability to carry and operate two Westland Whirlwinds from an aft deck and hangar, was to transform the capabilities of Antarctic patrol duties. It would also highlight very quickly the benefits of having Search and Rescue capabilities to hand in this geographically hostile area of the world.

Captain Michael Rawlinson OBE recalls his early flying years as a young Naval lieutenant (observer) operating Whirlwinds from HMS *Protector*. This would be his first journey into Antarctic waters and one that he would long remember:

We sailed Portsmouth on the 5th October 1956. This was to be HMS *Protector*'s second deployment for South Atlantic guard duties and Antarctic support. We arrived in Gibraltar on 9th October to refuel where we learnt with some concern that a group of Falkland Island Dependency Survey (FIDS) scientists with dogs were stranded on the Graham Land peninsula of Antarctica, due to an earlier than expected break-up of the surrounding sea ice. As we made our passage south we heard that the scientists had been located and all seemed well. However, on arrival at Rio de Janeiro on 28th October we received a signal that the FIDS team consisting of two men, their nine husky dogs and sledges were still stranded and now in danger and due to the melting ice unable to get to their base, Base W.

HMS *Protector* departed Rio immediately and made best speed for the Falklands, arriving in Port Stanley on the 4th November. We took on more fuel, stores and two relief scientists, and made last minute preparations for the rescue journey ahead. This included flying the two Whirlwind helicopters to a clear open space on Stanley Racecourse to recalibrate the aircraft compasses for accurate operating in southern latitudes.

Protector departed the Falklands as soon as possible and the flight used the passage south to gain operating experience in readiness for the demanding conditions in the Antarctic including rapidly changing wind and sea states and extremes in weather and visibility. Ice bergs became more frequent as we proceeded further south.

The exact whereabouts of the FIDS team was still uncertain. On the morning of Friday 9th November *Protector* arrived off the ice edge on the northwest of Adelaide Island, the weather was very poor and deck movement too excessive to

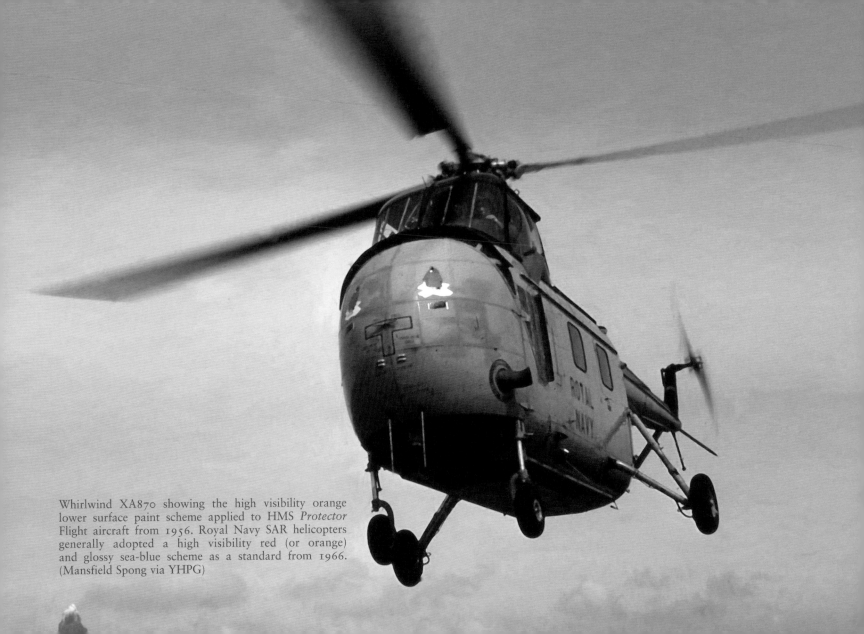

Whirlwind XA870 showing the high visibility orange lower surface paint scheme applied to HMS *Protector* Flight aircraft from 1956. Royal Navy SAR helicopters generally adopted a high visibility red (or orange) and glossy sea-blue scheme as a standard from 1966. (Mansfield Spong via YHPG)

consider attempting a reconnaissance flight. To compound matters one of the helicopters (XA 866) developed a fuel leak requiring a strip down and fuel tank change. The maintenance crew worked through the night to achieve this and at first light on the 10th November both aircraft were serviceable and ready for take-off. Deck conditions and the weather were much improved.

At 0610, Lieutenant John Brigham, the Flight CO and I as Observer took off in Whirlwind XA870 to search for the stranded FIDS team. Our maps and charts were limited for this region and were mostly outline coastal surveyor's charts and of limited help over the vast expanses of sea ice. However, an American Aeronautical map was a useful reminder of the high magnetic variation of 24 degrees east.

We had a rough idea of the location of the FIDS Base W and headed in that general direction. We took a visual reference of a prominent ice covered mountain outcrop and set the aircraft's gyro compass for a course to steer; the magnetic compass was unreliable. After about 30 minutes we were encouraged by making a visual sighting of what looked like the stranded team. On closing further we were able to report to Protector that we were over the stranded group and preparing to land and would probably be out of contact with the ship on losing height.

A low pass to assess the site revealed that the team were on the edge of a narrow ice shelf on Roux Island, with a sloping iced area to the front and steep rising bank behind. John made three different approaches to land but none were safe, the area being too small and confined. There were flat ice and snow covered surfaces close by but none appeared safe enough for a touchdown. We held off and circled the area while reconsidering a rescue plan. All the time we were burning valuable fuel and so decisions had to be made quickly in particular about how we were going to manage the dogs.

While circling we sighted the huts at Base W, a short flying distance away beyond a stretch of broken sea ice. It appeared to offer a better option for landing although again we had no idea how deep the snow would be. We decided that as a trial we would lift by winch one scientist and one dog and get them back to Base W. Depending on how that went we would decide if it were practical to ferry more than one dog at a time.

Lifting the scientist from the hover would be straight forward enough, but a large Husky dog was definitely going to be a first. We had no idea how the dog would respond to the confines of a noisy vibrating helicopter.

We had with us in the helicopter, on trial, a brand new hand held communications equipment known as TALBE (talk and listen beacon equipment). With a hastily scribbled 'how to use' note, it was lowered to the scientists. The equipment worked (!) and we were soon in voice contact with a team member, who agreed with the plan.

The lift would have to be made from a very low hover to keep the winching distance short, but not so low that the downdraft from the helicopter would create instant and dangerous white out conditions that could lead to disorientation; hazardous to both the helicopter and those below. As it was, John was having difficulty holding the helicopter close to the rising ground and over the ice ledge below.

The hoist of the one scientist, clutching a dog, went well considering the noise, the wind and swirling snow, as did the flight to the base camp with the scientist handler holding on to the dog the whole time. Base personnel had laid markers on the snow that provided some visual cues on the approach to landing. John made a number of approaches to assess the effect of blown snow. While in the final stage to land and at about five feet, in clouds of swirling snow the scientist, still clutching the dog, unexpectedly leapt from the helicopter! Fortunately it had snowed heavily the night before and they landed in a heap, in soft snow, without injury! Whether the jump was precipitated by the dog anxious to get out of the helicopter or the scientist I wasn't sure but clearly it was not a stunt to be repeated!

We had enough fuel to go back to Roux Island for another lift taking perhaps more than one dog this time. Over Roux and in the hover we could see that the handler was having problems with the next dog and those still on the traces were agitated. Seeing this plus the experience we had on the first transfer we realised we needed to stand off and consider other options.

Transferring one dog at a time, plus handler would take too long. The possibility of having a dog riot in the back of an airborne helicopter with a multi dog lift was not on either. It was clear that the dogs would have to be individually restrained as they came into the rear cabin.

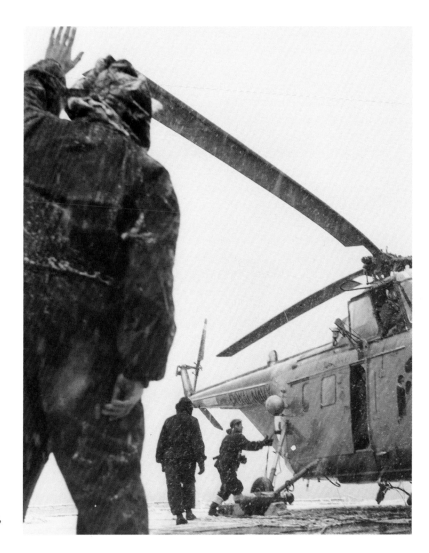

Preparing a Whirlwind helicopter for take-off on HMS *Protector*, 1960. Freezing temperatures and frozen deck conditions makes every task difficult, energy sapping and potentially dangerous. (FAA Museum)

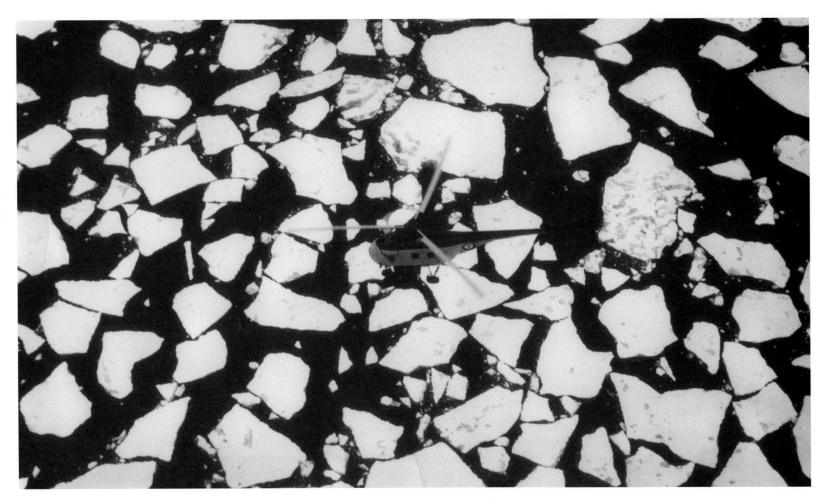

Extreme operating over Antarctic waters. There are very few suitable emergency landing zones in the Antarctic, so mechanics and maintainers must send the aircraft out 100 per cent reliable and fit to fly. (FAA Museum)

Having relayed this to the scientist and aware that we had now been airborne for a considerable time we needed to return to *Protector* to refuel. We had fuel in reserve; gauging fuel load and reserves is vitally important especially in ship board operations to allow for unforeseen circumstances or deteriorating weather en route, or on return, finding the deck 'fouled' necessitating a hold off while the deck was cleared.

Once at height we regained radio contact with the ship and reported progress plus that we would need some short lengths of line for the next flight. By the time we reached *Protector* we had been airborne for a total of 1 hour 50 minutes.

At 0845 after a quick turn round and some coffee Whirlwind XA870 was fuelled and ready. Now piloted by Lieutenant Mike Harvey we flew back to continue the rescue. Mike found the flight challenging as it was also his first experience of flying in extreme conditions where sky merged into ice often with no distinguishable features on horizon for reference. The ship had moved position since the first flight and the FIDS team were now about thirty five miles from the edge of the ice shelf and easier to relocate than on our first sortie. Using the TALBE the remaining scientist was told that we would do all the lifting again from a low hover, taking one dog first. As the husky came to the door opening I hauled it into the cabin and using the line secured the dog as closely as possible by its collar to the strengthening rail around the inside of the rear cabin. This worked well, if a bit undignified for the dog. Arriving over Base W, Mike like John, on the first sortie, made a number

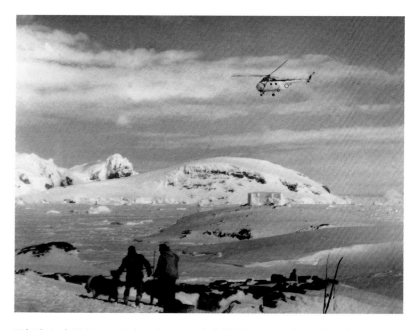

Whirlwind XA870 circles the stranded FIDS team while the pilot tries to identify a safe landing zone amid the snow drifts and ice ledges. (FAA Museum)

of approaches to assess the degree of blown snow. The scientist recalls that on the first Mike pulled away suddenly … swearing to himself … finally making an approach that limited the swirling snow sufficient to see enough to make a landing.

Taking the first scientist back to Roux we lifted another three dogs. Each lift took a little time and requiring precise flying. Holding the helicopter in position while doing this

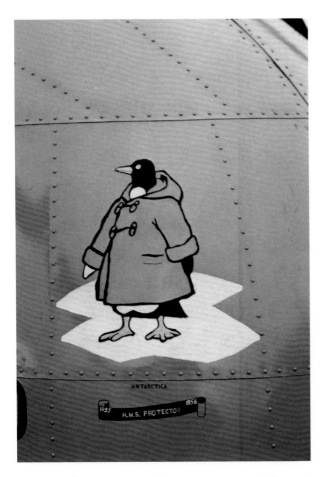

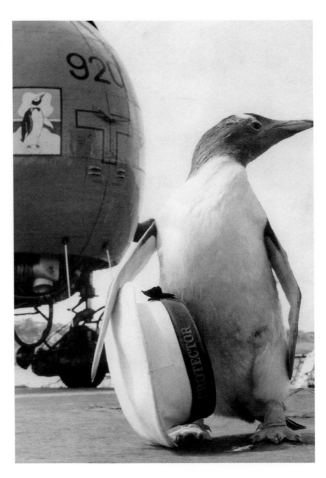

Close up of the *Protector* Flight's 'penguin in a duffle coat' emblem on the nose door of Whirlwind XA870 in 1956. Most *Protector* Flight aircraft have utilised some sort of penguin emblem ever since. (Mansfield Spong via YHPG)

Whirlwind XA866 (coded 920), HMS *Protector*, 1959. A different penguin emblem features on the helicopter nose doors, and a very willing real penguin temporarily joins the ship's company. (FAA Museum)

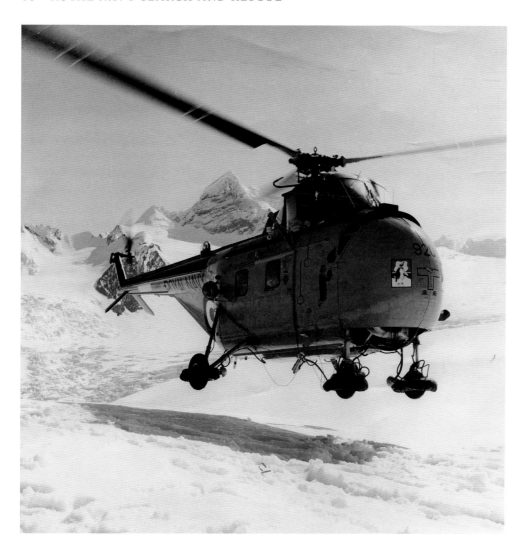

Whirlwind XA866 of HMS *Protector* pictured in a low hover at Royal Bay, South Georgia, in 1964. Note the aircraft's floatation devices attached to its wheels. In the event of an emergency water landing, these bags could be inflated (horizontally), rather like very large car inner tubes, to prevent the aircraft from sinking. (FAA Museum)

was quite a challenge for Mike who needed to break the hover briefly before coming in again to lift some of the scientific equipment. The transfer to the base went well, with the dogs now under better control. However, we hadn't enough fuel to safely lift the remaining dogs and sledges on that sortie and returned to *Protector* landing on at 1015.

The weather and steady deck conditions at ship contrasted markedly with the testing hovering required over the ice shelf and the hazardous blown snow conditions at the rescue site. At 1130, again in Whirlwind XA870 I returned with Mike to complete the rescue. We lifted and transferred three more dogs and a scientist then returning to the rescue site to hoist the remaining dog and with one of the scientists lifted the sledges and most of the remaining kit.

Meanwhile our other helicopter, XA866, appeared over the Base camp piloted by Lieutenant Brian Oliver delivering the two relief scientists and collecting some stores for return and their mail.

Landing safely back on *Protector* the whole rescue had taken around seven hours. It had been a very challenging and a memorable experience and one which clearly demonstrated the benefits and versatility of helicopter support from ships. The unpredictable nature of the weather was probably the greatest concern, it could change from blue skies and calm seas to a snow blizzard and pitching deck in minutes, very difficult to predict and very demanding conditions to operate in.

In the coming years Whirlwind helicopters from HMS *Protector* would conduct numerous Antarctic rescue and reconnaissance missions, including rescuing explorer Sir Edmund Hilary and his companion Dr Vivian Fuchs from a ship stranded in pack ice and struggling to make clear water. In this instance, Whirlwind XA870 was used to guide the ship on a path to the open sea, using its airborne position to great advantage. HMS *Protector* continued to regularly patrol the South Atlantic and Antarctic waters from 1955 until 1976, when she was replaced by HMS *Endurance* (equipped with Westland Wasp helicopters between 1976–1986 and Westland Lynx 1987–2008). Operating in a similar role of scientific and survey support while keeping a UK presence in the South Atlantic, the presence of HMS *Endurance* in this region would prove to be crucial for the Falkland Islands in the early 1980s.

While *Protector* Flight's Whirlwinds were operating in the sub-zero temperatures of the Antarctic, Royal Navy Whirlwind helicopters were busy in many other areas of the globe. One example of Navy helicopter support making a significant difference to life saving and assistance to shipping came from No. 845 NAS, attached to HMS *Bulwark* in the Gulf of Aden.

6

RESCUING PEOPLE – RESCUING SHIPS

On Saturday 13 September 1958, *Bulwark* received a signal that two oil tankers, *Ferdinand Gilabert* and *Melika*, had collided in the Arabian Sea. Both tankers were on fire and their respective crews had abandoned ship, but had been picked up by three other passing ships – *Border Hunter, Ceres* and *Anglian Diligence*. All crew were safe but many were badly injured or had sustained severe burns and neither of the passing ships had a doctor on board. HMS *Bulwark* altered course immediately and made ready three Whirlwind helicopters to transport naval doctors to the three ships. Having administered first aid treatment to the worst of the injured men, the helicopters transferred casualties and doctors back to *Bulwark* for further treatment. Later that afternoon, the nine most serious casualties were flown by helicopter to Masirah Island for further hospital treatment.

While the casualty evacuation was underway, two more Whirlwind helicopters were busy airlifting salvage parties onto the burning tankers in a bid to bring the blazing ships under control. The *Ferdinand Gilabert* was under control by the late afternoon, but it was well into the night before the fires on the *Melika* had been fully extinguished. The ships were clearly now a hazard to other

vessels and so it fell to HMS *Bulwark*, her crew and helicopter pilots to bring them into safety. At first light a towline was secured to the *Ferdinand Gilabert*, but due to the moderately rough sea conditions the towline parted, casting the ship adrift once more.

The morning of Sunday 14 September began with a series of ferry flights to both tankers delivering tools, pumps and all manner of other equipment needed to assist with stabilising the vessels and aid their recovery. Strong winds made the delivery of under-slung loads very difficult indeed as the helicopters moved in close to the now out-of-control ships to lower men and equipment. On Monday the 15th, a Whirlwind helicopter transferred a rope line between the *Melika* and HMS *Bulwark* which could be used to relay successive larger lines and cables between the two ships, until a 6 1/2-inch towing hawser could finally be secured between the two vessels. At this stage the *Melika* was finally brought under control, although at least one collision with the stern of *Bulwark* during the operation caused some damage to the aircraft carrier.

On Tuesday 16th, a succession of helicopter flights transferred more of *Bulwark*'s engineers and maintenance crew to the *Ferdinand Gilabert*, and later that day they were able to make

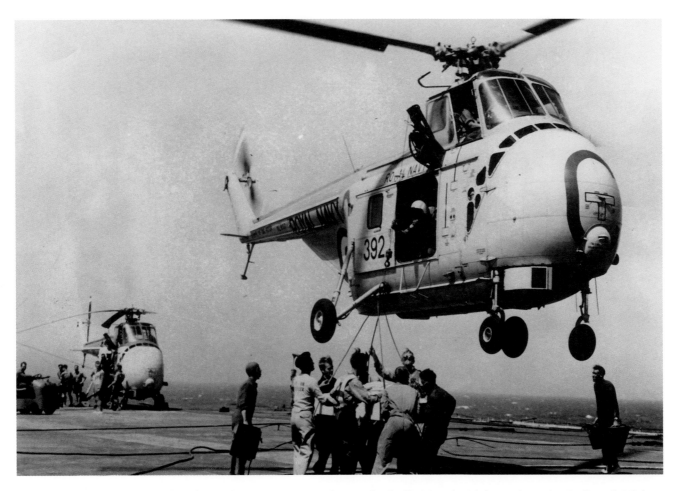

HMS *Bulwark* deck crews and medics rush to recover a merchant sailor badly injured with burns from the *Ferdinand Gilabert*. The casualty is being carried in an outboard stretcher box, probably because the helicopter was unable to land to take the casualty into the aircraft cabin. (FAA Museum)

her just capable of generating her own steam, and therefore did not need to be taken into tow.

The relentless routine of delivering maintenance crews, pumps, hoses, generators, barrels of diesel and other repair equipment continued many times a day, bringing with it a new problem for sustained winching operations in the field. The winch units were beginning to show signs of excessive use and needed repair and servicing. By Thursday 18th, all helicopter winching cables had been used beyond their serviceable limit and salvage party crews climbed hand-over-hand down a rope from the helicopter each time they went aboard the tankers, and used a rope ladder to return to the hovering helicopter. This very physically demanding and quite precarious practice was to continue regularly for another six days until the rescuing of the tankers was complete. The report in the squadron record book sums up the period of extraordinary flying. It reads:

> The rescue and salvage operation concerning the tankers *Melika* and *Ferdinand Gilabert* involved a total of 54 hours flying, 15 of which were casevacs or ferrying doctors to the injured. In the course of this flying 168 ferry trips were flown, 120 of these carrying every imaginable kind of load to and from the *Melika*. One load was lost due to premature release of the cargo hook. No required task was rejected as being impractical. As far as is known this was the first time helicopters have put salvage parties onboard an abandoned ship, let alone one on fire.

No. 845 NAS was subsequently awarded the Boyd Trophy for this outstanding feat of aviation and sustained flying in the assistance of the stricken vessels. This award, in the form of a solid silver

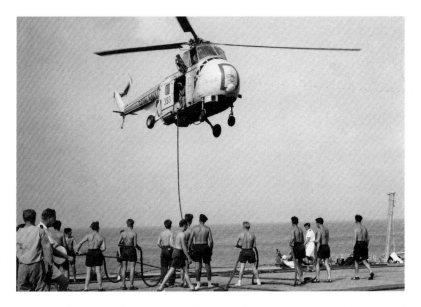

Whirlwind XK937 takes up a rope that is the first in a succession of connected lines and hawsers laid out on the deck of HMS *Bulwark*. This first line starts a sequence of passing successively larger towlines between *Bulwark* and the stricken vessel *Melika*, culminating in the transfer of the final 6-inch diameter towing hawser. (FAA Museum)

model of a Fairey Swordfish, is presented by Flag Officer Naval Air Command annually to any ship or squadron who has carried out a remarkable flying achievement in that last year.

Finally ending service in 1976 after nearly twenty-five years, the Whirlwind had held its own alongside the more modern Wessex and Wasp helicopter types during this period. It will hold a place in the memories of many, not least those that owe their lives to it from a successful rescue.

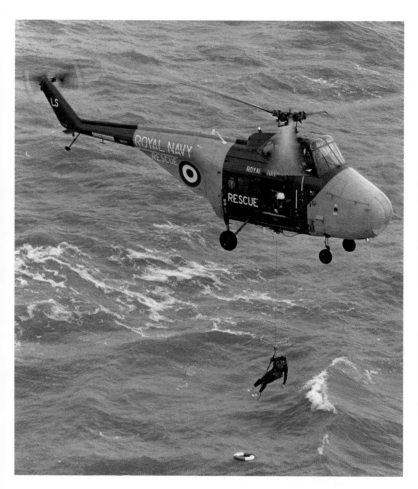

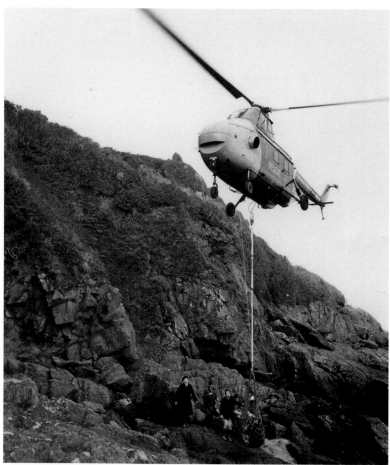

SAR crews practice as often as possible to remain familiar with, and to develop new, procedures and techniques. Constant practice, even with basic 'wet winching' exercises, keeps the team honed to perfection. (FAA Museum)

SAR comes in all shapes and sizes. Whirlwind XN306 is pictured again here, operating from RNAS Brawdy Station Flight and performing a live cow rescue from the cliffs in west Wales. (FAA Museum)

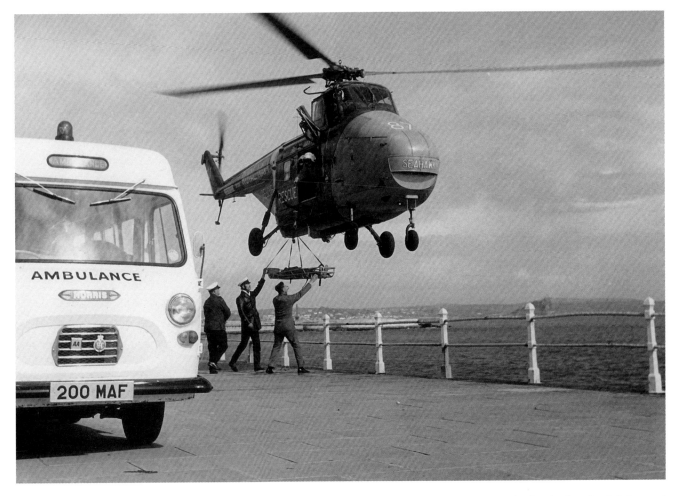

Whirlwind XN306 from RNAS Culdrose during a casevac stretcher exercise on Penzance promenade. Precise low-level flying and hovering is the daily 'norm' for a Royal Navy SAR pilot. (FAA Museum)

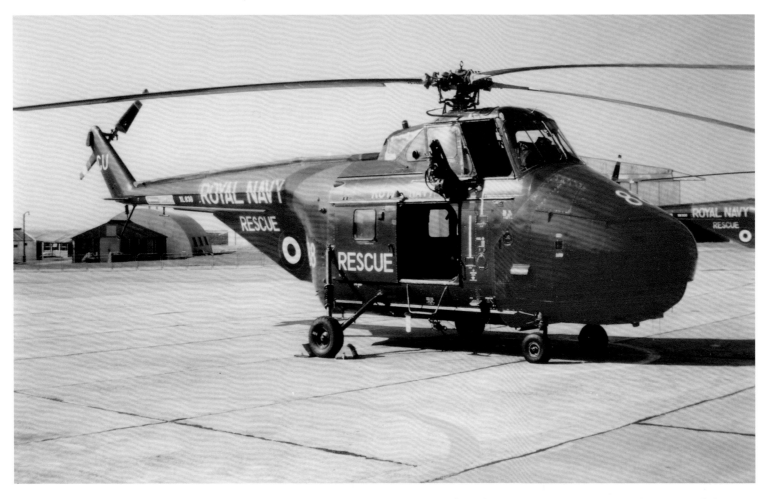

Whirlwind HAR 9 showing the bright signal-red and glossy sea-blue scheme that was adopted as a standard scheme on Royal Navy SAR helicopters from 1966. (FAA Museum)

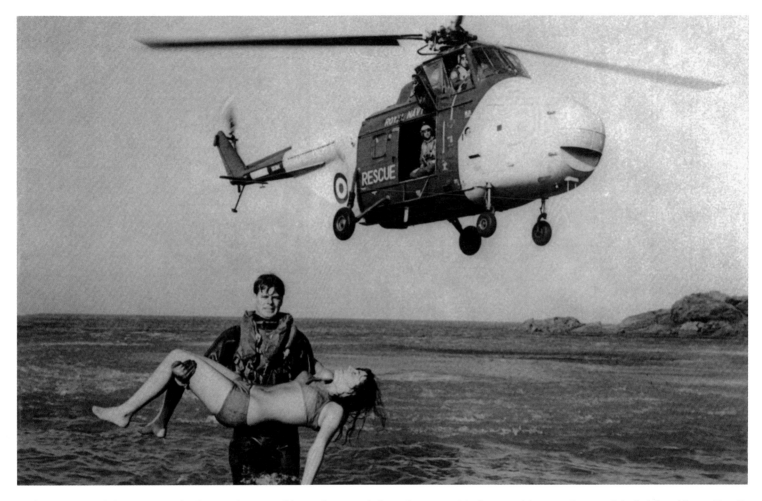

A classic, and slightly tongue-in-cheek, Royal Navy publicity photograph from the 1970s. It's the age of the superhero and the height of James Bond's popularity, but the message is clear – when it comes to SAR, the Royal Navy will go to the limit to save you. (MOD Copyright 2014)

7

WESTLAND WESSEX

It is normal for new aircraft types to be introduced into service while a previous type is still performing an active role. This ensures continuity and allows for a trial, development and handover period to be undertaken. In 1958, with the Whirlwind having been in service for only five years, Britain saw the arrival of yet another Sikorsky design (the S.58), again licence-built by the Westland company and called the Wessex. The Wessex was powered by the new Napier Gazelle gas turbine engine and was the first helicopter to be fitted from the factory with an auto-pilot system, making night flying an easier task than before.

Capable of carrying up to twelve people (in addition to the crew), or (in good weather conditions) 1 ton of under-slung load, this new type would again set new benchmarks for helicopter operation and capability. All Wessex Mks used by the Royal Navy (Mk 1, Mk 3 and Mk 5) were capable of and frequently used for SAR duties.

By the 1960s, the Wessex 1 was operating with no fewer than ten Royal Navy squadrons around the world. Following the troubles in Malaya between 1948 and 1960, tensions in Borneo meant that British forces remained in this area of South East Asia to continue to stabilise the situation. During this period the Wessex Mk1 began to take over from the Whirlwind and would show its worth many times over as a jungle warfare support helicopter, general workhorse and, of course, very capable SAR helicopter.

Reports from No. 845 NAS's record book in September 1964 clearly show that no fewer than sixty-seven casevacs (casualty evacuations) had been carried out in a single month. The record concludes by stating that 'no call for a casevac was turned down by the squadron and all missions were successfully completed. Medical evidence indicates that many of those casevaced would otherwise have died'.

One extraordinary mission involved the rescue of a fifteen-year-old Iban native boy called Kumbang, who had sustained an incredibly serious head injury. The accident happened at about 4.30 p. m. on 19 September 1964. Mr John Wilson, Rural Development Officer stationed in the Nanga Entabai region of Borneo, had an emergency message that the boy needed most

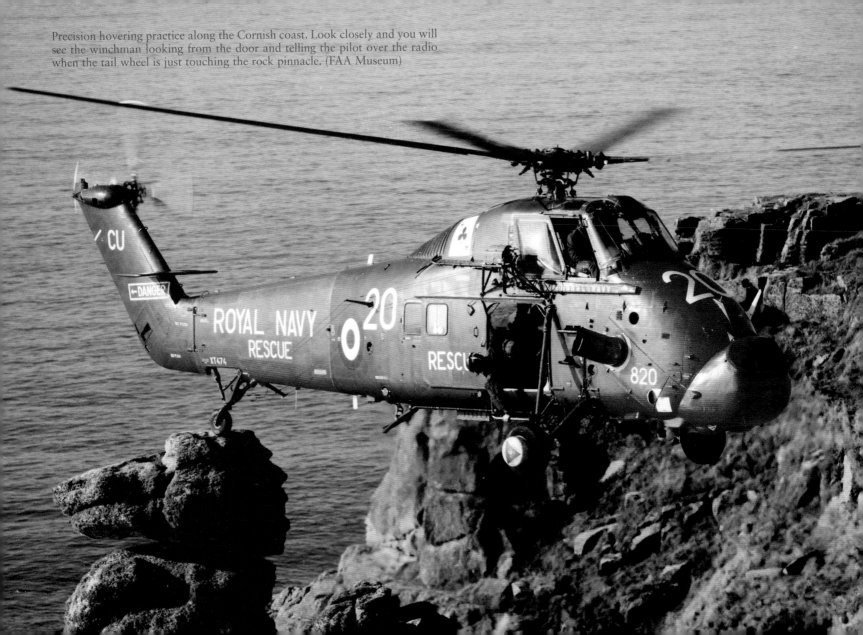

Precision hovering practice along the Cornish coast. Look closely and you will
see the winchman looking from the door and telling the pilot over the radio
when the tail wheel is just touching the rock pinnacle. (FAA Museum)

urgent hospital treatment if he were to live. Mr Wilson (himself a former RAF Wing Commander) immediately started to try and make radio contact with No. 845 NAS, which he knew was based some 30 miles to the north. However, the weather was poor and torrential rain and poor atmospherics meant that it was nearly eight o'clock before successful communications were established and a helicopter dispatched to collect the casualty. It was now dark and the rain was still pouring down, certainly not ideal conditions to attempt a night flight across jungle territory to a small makeshift landing zone among high trees. But there was a life at stake, and No. 845 Squadron were probably the last hope. Duty Pilot Lt Kennard, along with observer Lt MacPherson and winchman/aircrewman Petty Officer Smith, gave the thought of a night flight over jungle terrain much consideration, but elected to give it a go if a young boy was in grave danger.

Navigating over jungle landscape at night in driving rain is difficult and problematic enough, particularly in a single engine helicopter, but landing in a makeshift clearing among the trees is incredibly dangerous. The Wessex was equipped with a powerful downward-facing search-and-landing spotlight, which would be fairly useful in normal night conditions. However, in driving jungle rain, the light was considered to be almost no use at all as all it did was illuminate a screen of windblown rain and spray, making accurate positioning on the descent very difficult indeed. But with some highly skilled flying by Lt Kennard, a safe

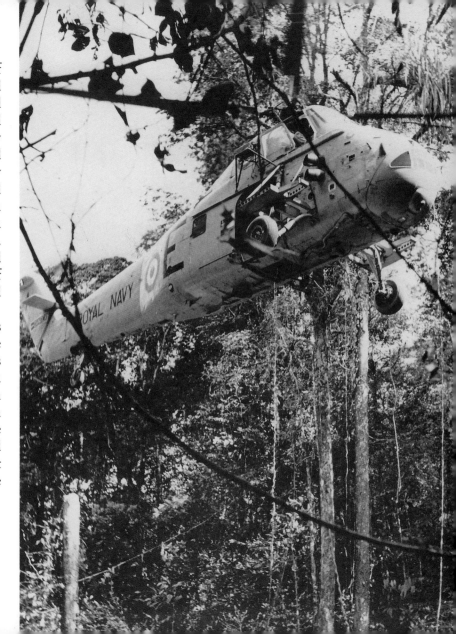

Jungle operational flying, this time in Borneo, and Wessex XP108 makes a confined area landing among the trees. Providing that it can find a suitable place to land, a helicopter can rescue a casualty in an hour where it would otherwise take several days on foot. (FAA Museum)

landing was achieved. Mr Wilson later stated that the weather conditions were so poor that had an Aldis signal lamp been available, he would have signalled to the pilot, 'many thanks for mercy attempt – but advise no attempt at landing'.

On the ground, and after such an arduous flight, the helicopter crew were initially frustrated to see the patient being assisted to walk (albeit gingerly) from the field hospital towards the helicopter. Had they just risked their lives and a helicopter for a patient that could walk? As the casualty came closer, their frustration turned to disbelief as they could see in the gloom that the young boy had a fishing spear piercing his head, with a portion of the thin harpoon sticking some twelve inches out from each side. The spear had gone through a frontal part of the skull in about the only precise area where surviving such an injury would be possible.

The gravity of the situation now struck home and thoughts turned to getting him into the helicopter without jarring the spear in the doorway, and how to transport him as comfortably as possible in a helicopter with a vibration level that was significant, to say the least. Again, with some extremely skilled piloting the crew managed to transport the boy as swiftly and smoothly as possible back to 845's base at Sibu. Back at base the emergency ambulance crew were similarly frustrated at the thought of having raced out in the night to collect a walking patient. They, too, were stopped in their tracks when the full extent of the injury could be assessed, not least by their having to open both ambulance doors to carefully get the young man in.

Miraculously, the boy survived an operation to remove the spear and was returned sometime later to his family longhouse at Nanga Entabai.

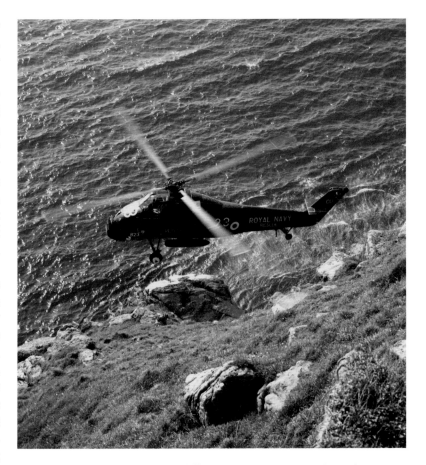

When people get stranded on a cliff ledge you can't rescue them if you can't get close. Regular practice makes this extremely dangerous close cliff flying an essential discipline. The pilot is in the right-hand seat, so flying with the rotor blades nearest the cliff face on his blind side is a very difficult manoeuvre indeed. (FAA Museum)

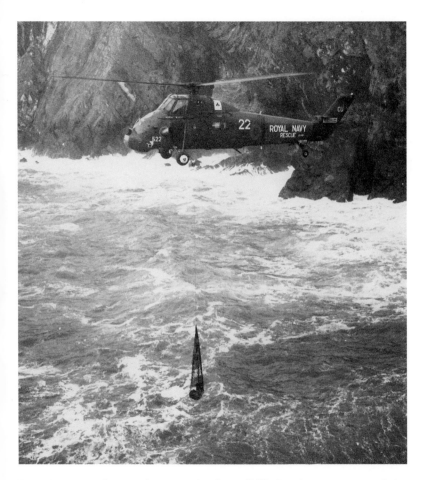

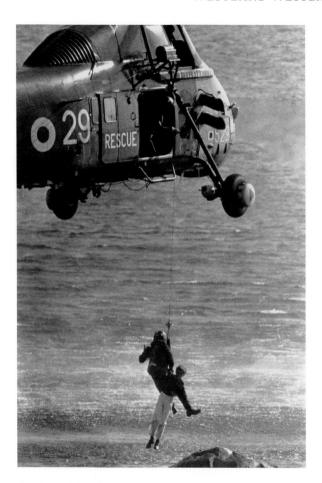

Rescuing cows, sheep and even ponies from cliff ledges is a common task for Navy SAR crews. Clearly No. 771 Squadron expect to perform a number of these each year. Their record book entry for 8 January 1982 reads: 'First cow lift of 1982!' (FAA Museum)

Why precision hovering is so important. A Wessex of No. 771 Squadron rescuing the second of two small boys stranded on a rock by a swift incoming tide at Mount's Bay, Cornwall, in 1976. (FAA Museum/*Cornish Photo News*).

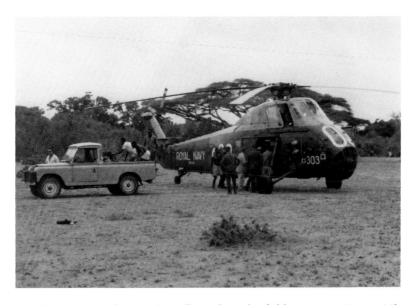

A different kind of rescue but all good 'in the field' practice. Wessex Mk I helicopter from HMS *Ark Royal* assists in the rescue of a colony of rare Hunter's hartebeest in Kenya, airlifting the crated animals (appropriately) two-by-two to a new, safe environment. (FAA Museum)

In a letter to the Squadron Commander of No. 845 Naval Air Squadron, Mr Wilson states:

I do not know who the pilot was, but he did carry out a splendid night landing under very, very difficult conditions and evacuated the patient. I consider the action one of great bravery, determination and courage which should not go unmentioned and I would be grateful if you would give this

incident a special mention. We know that pilots and crew treat these things as part of their work but he would have been well within his rights had he decided not to land.

No photographs appear to exist of the incident, but it is believed that the spear was presented to No. 845 Squadron by the surgeon as a most unusual squadron trophy!

During its long career the Wessex type helicopter would be involved in a vast range of tasks, from run-of-the-mill plane guard duties alongside aircraft carriers, to some of the most diverse and hazardous flying duties imaginable.

Among the more unusual was the rescue of a colony of rare antelope in Africa. Most people would normally associate a rescue mission being confined to the safe recovery of a small number of human beings, but helping to rescue an entire sub-species of animal from extinction is certainly out of the ordinary. However, in October 1963 this is exactly what was requested of the helicopter crews of No. 815 Naval Air Squadron.

The squadron was embarked in HMS *Ark Royal* when it received a signal requesting assistance from the Kenyan government to help move to a safe enclosure as many as possible of the last known herd of Hunter's hartebeest. These particular hartebeest were trapped on land that was to undergo a vast irrigation and development programme. In addition to that, the autumn rains would present a slim chance of survival for the animals on what would remain of their territory. The Tsavo Royal National Park had identified a safe game reserve some eighty miles north of the area, but transferring some antelope by earlier attempts was proving too difficult. A road trip was too rough and was taking too long; some of the early moves had overstressed the antelope and a few had died as a result. Air lifting using an RAF Pioneer cargo aircraft was little better, with a lengthy transport time to the airstrip and bumpy take-off and landing again proving too much for many of the delicate animals. A short heli-lift direct from the capture pens to the release zone was thought to be the only solution and with approval from the Admiralty, HMS *Ark Royal* detailed No. 815 NAS to respond.

With a narrow window of opportunity before the autumn rains set in (making the task unachievable), ground crews, engineers and refuelling crews were flown by helicopter into a forward operating position near to the captured hartebeest.

The operation would have to be slick and it was imperative that the animals were moved as quickly as possible from A to B and with minimum of waiting time.

Take offs and landings would have to be as smooth as possible. Putting the animals into specially designed darkened crates would need to be done swiftly and with the aircraft ready to go. There was no room for error and crews would have to keep a very tight timetable of refuelling and maintenance checks to ensure the helicopters would not go un-serviceable with a load half prepared, which could prove fatal to the live cargo.

The receiving end would need to be similarly prepared and be ready to receive and deal with releasing the animals and monitoring their condition while they waited for the next batch. It was found that three crates could be fitted into the rear cargo area of the Wessex, and that with enough normal service equipment stripped out it would still be within the operational weight limit of the helicopter. Of course there was only a limited number of crates, and each delivery would have to await the release of the animals so that the helicopter could return with the empty crates for reloading. The turnaround time at each end took about one hour, so during a typical day's flying the two helicopters on task could make two trips each, transporting the antelope two at a time, and with an occasional trip of three. There was not sufficient daylight to safely perform a third trip each day. Take-off and landing was particularly hazardous and downwash from the helicopter rotor blades would stir up a thick cloud of fine red dust which would envelope the helicopter, making clear visual reference with the ground all but impossible. Extremely skilled and steady flying was required to ensure that the helicopter took off, landed safely and in a manner that was smooth enough so as not to stress or alarm the animals on board. After two days' flying, the twenty hartebeest that had been captured had successfully been transported to the safe reserve, and with the onset of heavy rain on Saturday 26 October, Operation Antelope was brought to a close. As an expression of gratitude for saving the hartebeest, *Ark Royal* was made an honorary life member of the East African Wildlife Society.

One might ask the question as to why a military service should get itself involved in so many varied scenarios, and at what justification of cost? The answer to that is twofold. Firstly, you only get good at flying and operating logistically in difficult and demanding situations by actually doing it – it is certainly not something that can be learned in the classroom, with the hope of being able to do it for real when the time comes. All of the things that are experienced and learned from the endless variety of requests to get someone or something out of danger are in themselves a rolling programme of continual training that allows the pilots and support crews to hone their skills and learn

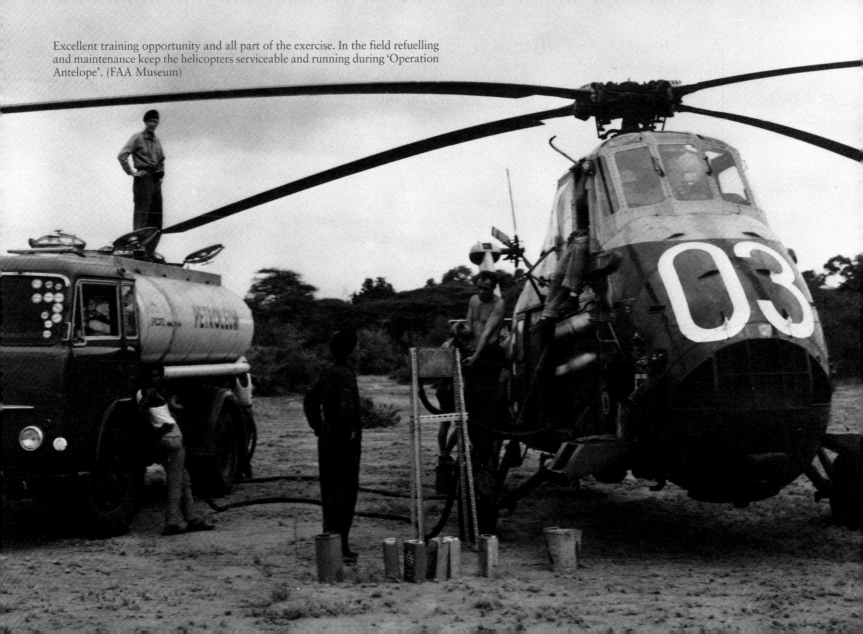

Excellent training opportunity and all part of the exercise. In the field refuelling and maintenance keep the helicopters serviceable and running during 'Operation Antelope'. (FAA Museum)

to deal with extreme situations. Who knows when they may need to draw on a particular experience or lesson learned when operating in a battlefield situation? Such varied flying helps to prepare pilots and crews for just about anything, and enables them to pass on vast amounts of knowledge and experience to the next generation of airmen, engineers and field support teams. Secondly, there are also many instances where winning the hearts and minds of those around you, particularly in foreign countries or waters, is extremely valuable and can make a great deal of difference in the general role of peacekeeping and developing friendly borders around the globe.

Winter Emergencies

Winter conditions in Great Britain are thankfully not normally too severe. However, occasionally there have been extreme spells of heavy snow and sustained freezing temperatures that have made daily operating a significant challenge throughout the country. In the winter of 1962/63, there was a particularly heavy and prolonged period of snow, and again during the 1970s there were several winters that brought the country to a standstill, caught out by extreme weather.

Under such conditions emergency situations begin to show up very quickly – people snowbound and stranded in cars, the severely ill and the elderly needing specialist and regular medical treatment or supplies and the transporting of basic food stuffs to collection points become essential and immediate tasks. In some districts, power lines may also have been brought down by the weight of snow, causing widespread communication problems.

The emergency services can only do so much with their normal modes of transport, and the armed forces are usually ready to assist with both manpower and specialist equipment where necessary. One area where the Royal Navy can contribute is with helicopter support to assist with critical transport needs. Ordinarily it might only be the Search and Rescue squadrons who would be tasked for such activities, but when the problem becomes a nationwide emergency situation, then Commando squadrons and training squadrons may also be drafted in to increase support. However, this is not without its problems, as many of the squadron's crews may be living 'ashore' (the Navy term for living away from the main air base) and also amid the now cut off and isolated communities. In such instances squadron personnel may have to trudge miles through snowbound roads and lanes to return to their units.

Of direct benefit to the immediate communities and the nation as a whole, this valuable work also provides an unexpected Arctic training exercise, with very real learning experiences for the squadron crews and very real outcomes for those in need of emergency assistance.

Some human and animal lives are sadly lost as a result of extreme winter weather, but many more are saved thanks to the skill and determination of all the national services that do what they can to save lives and help keep the country functioning in time of need.

Desperate situations sometimes call for desperate measures, and occasionally the rule book may not be as closely observed as it should be.

Lt Mike Smith was a Royal Navy Lt Pilot in May 1966, flying Wessex helicopters in Borneo. No. 848 Naval Air Squadron were

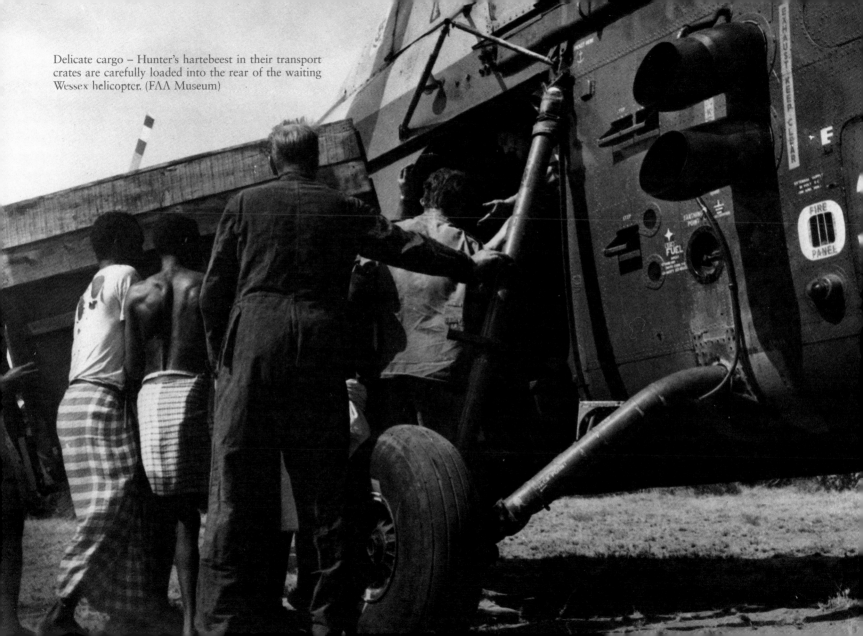

Delicate cargo – Hunter's hartebeest in their transport crates are carefully loaded into the rear of the waiting Wessex helicopter. (FAA Museum)

operating alongside other British armed forces in the region as part of the stabilisation force and also assisting the Geographical Survey Department in accurately mapping the country. Mike recalls:

Our daily tasking was ferrying food, ammunition, medical supplies etc. to various jungle locations in support of the troops on the ground. This was pretty challenging in itself as much of the area was not accurately mapped, so in many instances we were flying over vast areas of jungle with very scant reference to exactly where we were. Many of our maps and charts simply ran out of detail in some areas, and we were using handed down maps from our predecessors, No. 845 Squadron, with hand-drawn reference points, mountains, rivers etc. These were pretty good, but all very locally produced!

During this time, we had a signal to say that a section of Parachute Regiment troops were stranded in the jungle, near the Indonesian border and about 100 miles away from our base at Nanga-Gaat. Of the ten-man section, we were told that at least five of them had sustained serious injuries whilst on patrol. Two or three had bad fevers, one had fallen badly and broken his pelvis, and another had a sustained a bad knife wound whilst trying to hack through the undergrowth. Clearly they were not going to make 100 miles on foot through the jungle.

They did have a basic location beacon, and we went out late in the afternoon to overfly the area and see if we could trace them. After about an hour we got a basic reading on the locator, but the best we could do was narrow their position down to approximately two to three hundred yard radius. This was just not good enough and the jungle canopy was so full and thick that it was impossible to peer down into the dark jungle and get any positive visual on the men. It was also getting dark and we were low on fuel, so we headed to a Ghurkha base about fifteen miles south and landed there for the night. Next day we set out again and

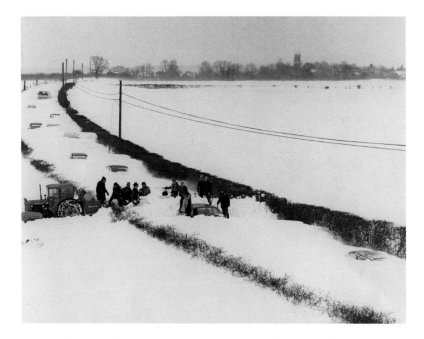

Image taken from the doorway of a Royal Navy helicopter as the crew surveys stranded cars amid the snow drifts near to RNAS Yeovilton during the winter of 1976. (FAA Museum)

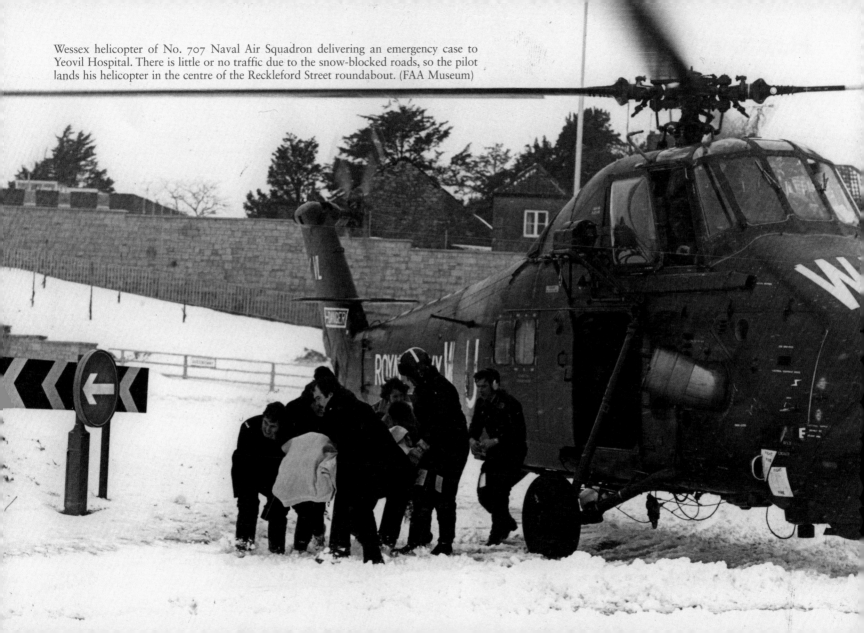

Wessex helicopter of No. 707 Naval Air Squadron delivering an emergency case to Yeovil Hospital. There is little or no traffic due to the snow-blocked roads, so the pilot lands his helicopter in the centre of the Reckleford Street roundabout. (FAA Museum)

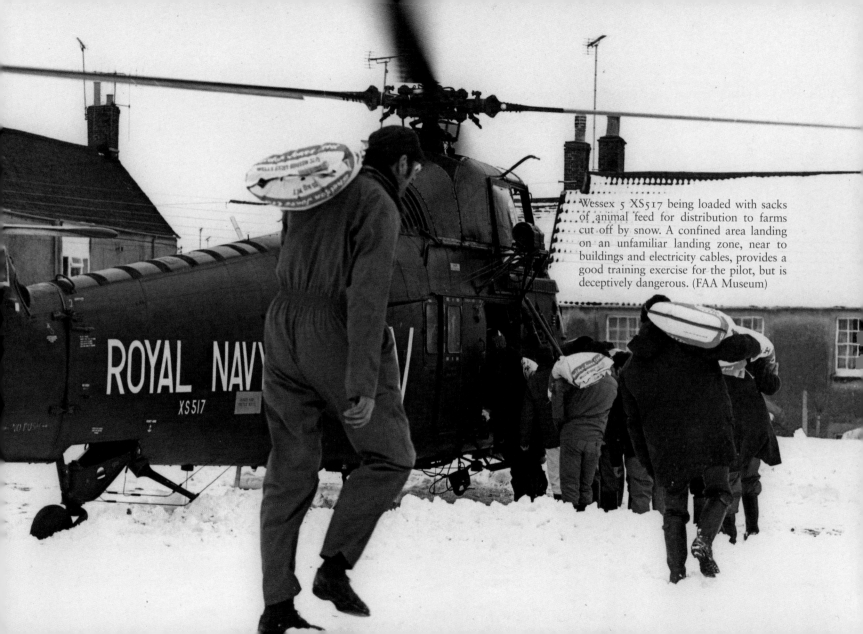

Wessex 5 XS517 being loaded with sacks of animal feed for distribution to farms cut off by snow. A confined area landing on an unfamiliar landing zone, near to buildings and electricity cables, provides a good training exercise for the pilot, but is deceptively dangerous. (FAA Museum)

Winter 1976, and cattle look on bemused as No. 771 Search and Rescue Squadron deliver vital feed supplies. Even when snow was receding in some areas, many road systems remained blocked, necessitating helicopter support from Naval Air Squadrons. (FAA Museum)

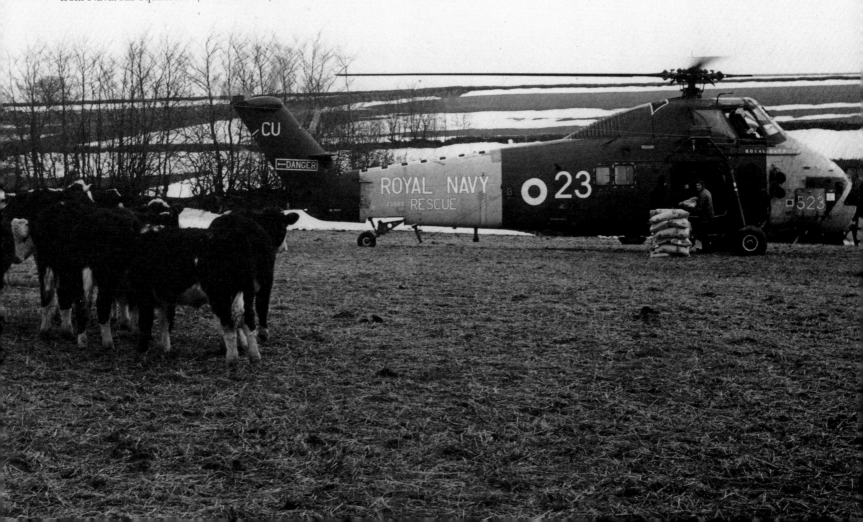

found our best position with the beacon. We then let down our aircrew/winchman on the full extent of cable, which was ninety feet, and lowered him to the top of the tree canopy as close to the beacon area as possible. He did make a visual contact with the troops, but the trees were so tall that he was still about 150 feet short of reaching them.

We returned to the Ghurkha camp and re-thought the plan. We would need to land to pick up and evacuate the injured troops, but to do that we would have to get down onto the jungle floor and clear a suitable area, using explosive charges to clear some trees. I measured the rope on the helicopter message lowering bag and at 150 feet decided that if this was attached to the end of the winch wire, we might just have enough line to get someone onto the jungle floor.

It was highly dangerous and way outside of the rules, so I decided that I had better volunteer myself rather than subject my winchman to my crazy idea, I would also need a skilful winch operator in the helicopter. My co-pilot David Baston agreed to fly me, and so the plan was set.

What you have to remember here is that the message bag rope could not be wound onto the winch line drum, so we had to tie it to the end of the winch line and David flew me hanging on a rope 150 feet below the helicopter for fifteen miles across the jungle to get back to the stranded troops. At that point our winchman started to lower me the remaining ninety feet of cable length down through the canopy among the thicket of leaves and branches. This was extremely dangerous and required great skill from David to keep the helicopter in a steady hover or I would have been badly injured myself among the tree branches. With the winch cable fully out, and me now way out of sight down among the undergrowth, I was still not on the jungle floor. Until the winch cable went slack and I could give it a series of tugs to signal my safe decent, only then could they withdraw the winch line and stand-off with the helicopter at a safe distance.

David realised this and in an attempt to gain me what he hoped would be the critical few extra feet, he very carefully nestled the helicopter down into the uppermost branches of the trees. Again, this was a highly dangerous manoeuvre and the helicopter did receive some light damage to the underside skins, but it worked! I was on the floor and quickly removed my harness. I took the harness off the rope so that it would not snag in the branches, gave the signal to pull up and the helicopter flew away to a safe distance.

With help from a couple of the uninjured paras, we set charges around a selection of trees and in a short space of time had cleared a zone big enough to allow David to bring the Wessex down into a very confined space landing area. We bundled everyone on board, pulled up and headed back to Nanga-Gaat, where we could get the troops the urgent medical treatment that they needed. We had done it by the skin of our teeth, but it was obvious from the condition of the injured troops that some of them would not have made another day and night in the jungle.

The Wessex helicopter would prove itself time and time again as a dependable SAR helicopter. From rescuing fishermen and yachtsmen in dangerous seas, to extracting stranded holiday

Lt Mike Smith at the Controls of a No. 848 Squadron Wessex 5 Helicopter in Borneo, 1966. (FAA Museum)

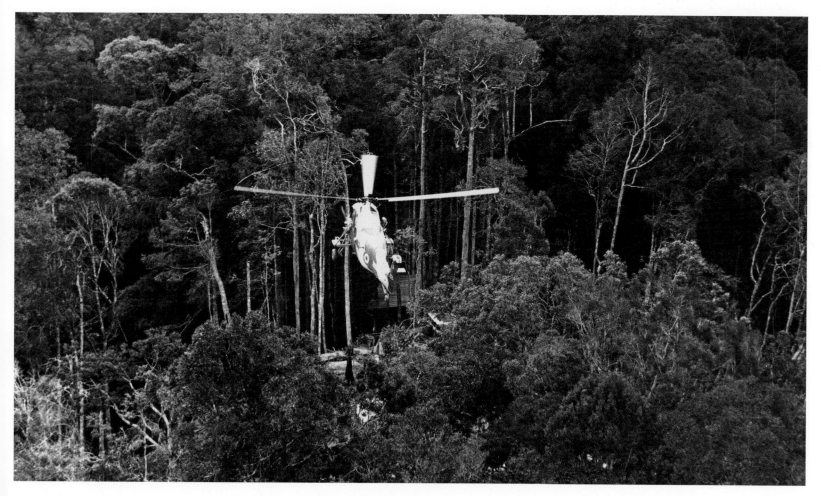

A No. 848 Squadron Wessex 5 over the Borneo jungle in the 1960s. No photographs exist of Lt Mike Smith's daring rescue, but this image describes well the tricky situation both he and his pilot had to negotiate to reach the stranded British troops some 200 feet beneath the tree canopy. (FAA Museum)

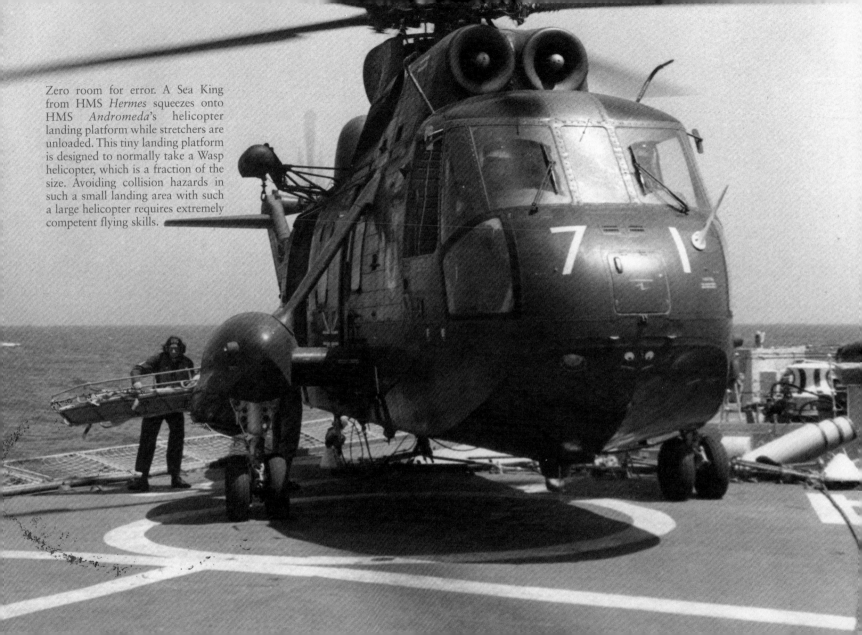

Zero room for error. A Sea King from HMS *Hermes* squeezes onto HMS *Andromeda*'s helicopter landing platform while stretchers are unloaded. This tiny landing platform is designed to normally take a Wasp helicopter, which is a fraction of the size. Avoiding collision hazards in such a small landing area with such a large helicopter requires extremely competent flying skills.

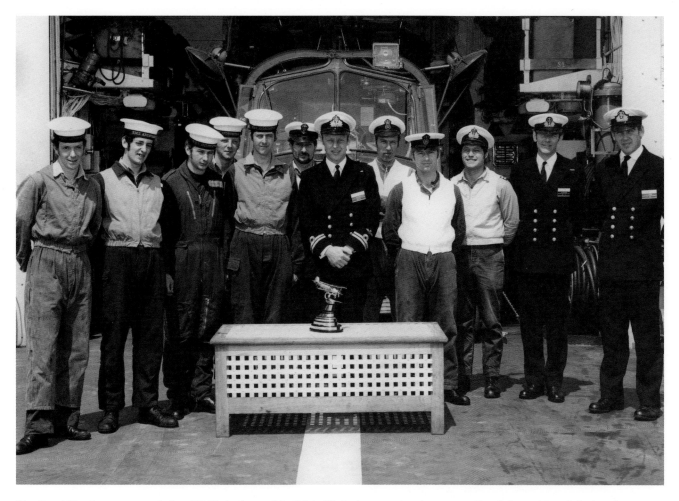

The Boyd Trophy was awarded to HMS *Andromeda*'s Ship's Flight in 1974 for the outstanding flying achieved during the rescues off Cyprus that year. Lt McKechnie (centre) with some of the ship's flight crew, in front of Wasp XT421. (FAA Museum)

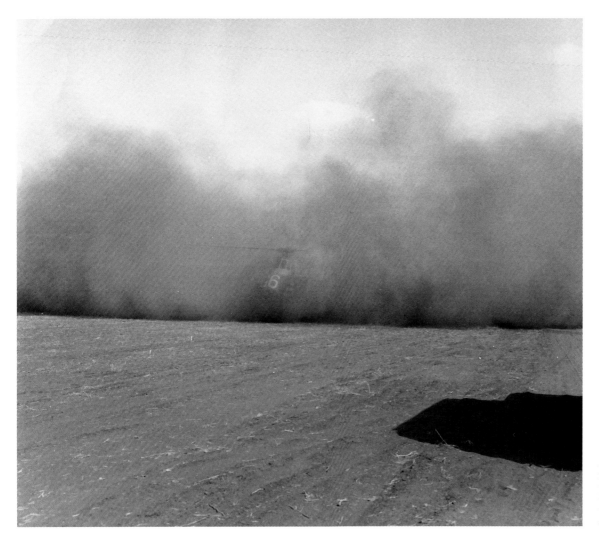

Instrument flying in dust storm conditions. Delivering the rescued hartebeest to their new safe National Park location involved take offs and landings amid swirling clouds of red sand dust. (FAA Museum)

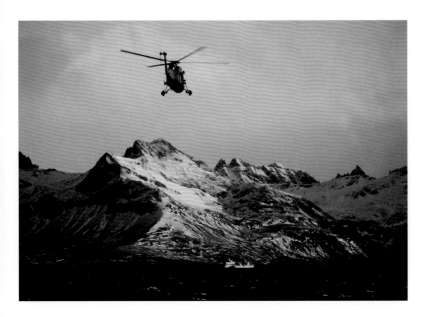

Wessex XP142 *Humphrey* sets out towards Fortuna Glacier, South Georgia. (FAA Museum)

makers from cliff ledges or tidal reefs; lifting animals to safety or delivering food stuffs to snowbound villages; racing patients with urgent medical needs to hospital, to plucking injured workmen from the tops of tall buildings: the Wessex has done them all and more.

Using helicopters to insert or recover troops from battlefield situations is a standard task, with many helicopters being specifically designed and equipped. However, during the Falklands Campaign in 1982, Royal Navy crews operating a

Mk 3 Wessex helicopter equipped for anti-submarine work would execute one of the most amazing SAR missions on record.

Argentinian movements in the South Atlantic needed to be watched in great detail as tension in the region escalated. Reports of Argentinian forces occupying Grytviken, on South Georgia, prompted the British military to airlift sixteen SAS troops onto the glacier over-looking the area and observe Argentinian movements around the areas of Leith and Stromness Bay.

The route to the top of Fortuna Glacier would have to be from the north side, flying in low over Possession Bay and Antarctic Bay before beginning the difficult flight up through the mountains to a landing zone on top of the glacier.

The SAS troops and their equipment would be carried in two Commando support Wessex 5s from RFA *Tidespring*, while Wessex 3, XP142 from HMS *Antrim*, would lead the way. Wessex XP142, affectionately nick-named *Humphrey*, would use its anti-submarine radar, normally configured to read and map underwater objects and terrain, to read the treacherous mountain valleys and crevasses and allow the convoy of three helicopters to thread their way low and close through the mountain passes to the drop off point.

The three helicopters set off at daybreak on 21 April, but low cloud, thick fog and driving rain near the mountains forced a return to the ship. By early afternoon conditions had improved a little and it was decided to try again. Visibility was still difficult and the ascent to the top of Fortuna Glacier tested all three pilots to the limit, experiencing swirling cloud, rain, snow and sudden changes in wind speed and direction. Having made the landing zone and decanted the troops and equipment, the three helicopters then had to thread their way back down through the ravines and valleys of the mountain to avoid detection. The mission had so far been a success but nightfall would bring a new twist to the episode.

The weather deteriorated further, with a huge drop in temperature and Storm Force 10 gales blasting onto the mountainside. The ship's report for the day notes that the SAS on the glacier had radioed to say that 'their position had become untenable and that they believed they would have difficulty surviving another twelve hours up there'.

It was time to get them out, and it would be *Humphrey* who would quite literally save the day.

All three helicopters refuelled and set off in formation as before, following *Humphrey* low across Possession Bay for the ascent at the rear of the mountain. Conditions were significantly worse than the previous day with wind speeds rising and falling from anything between 10 knots and 70 knots, bringing with it snow and swirling cloud. It was decided that the two Commando Wessexes would touch down on a spit of land between Possession Bay and Antarctic Bay to conserve fuel, while *Humphrey* continued on up the glacier, using its radar to assess conditions at the top. However, after three attempts to do so, conditions were deemed to be so bad that all three helicopters had to return to their respective ships to refuel and await a lull in the weather. Time was now against the whole operation and daylight was fading fast. After the briefest of refuels, the three helicopters set off again and through sheer determination and skilled airmanship managed to reach the top of the glacier. Hearing the helicopters coming through the mist and swirling cloud, the SAS troops lit a smoke flare to signal the position of a safe landing zone. A brief gap in the weather allowed the helicopters to land and be swiftly loaded with troops and equipment. As the last men climbed aboard, the weather closed in again. High winds created vast swirling snow clouds, causing complete white-out conditions. Lt Mike Tidd, flying the Wessex coded 'A', lifted and began to transition forward into flight, but almost immediately became disorientated within the featureless white-out surrounding him. He lost control of his helicopter, causing it to crash onto its side in a snow bank about 50 yards away from the others. Fortunately, he had not gained much height or speed and apart from some small injuries no one was seriously hurt. The remaining two helicopters lifted successfully and having checked their own weight and handling, moved forward and settled again near to the crashed Wessex. Both *Humphrey* and the second Wessex, coded 'F', dumped fuel to offset the extra weight and between them crammed the troops and equipment from the crashed Wessex onboard. Visibility was virtually nil and the weather conditions still severe, but there was nowhere to stay on the mountain. *Humphrey* took off with Wessex 'F' following line astern as closely as possible, trying desperately not to lose sight of the lead ship with its terrain following radar. The two very over-laden helicopters were now making their way precariously down the glacier. As they approached a small ridge, *Humphrey* managed to crest it safely, but disastrously Wessex 'F', without the advantage of on-board radar, struck the ridge and crashed onto its side. This was now very serious. Not only was there no radio contact from Wessex 'F', but *Humphrey*, considerably overloaded and short of fuel (having jettisoned some to reduce weight), was committed to returning to HMS *Antrim*, leaving behind a completely unknown situation in the swirling blizzard.

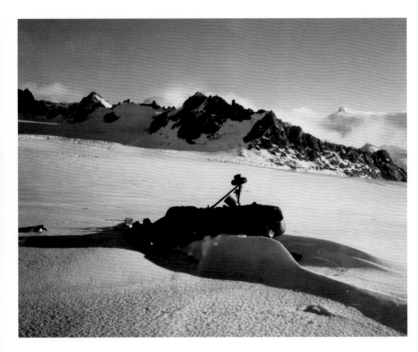

Right: Safe back on HMS *Antrim*, the Special Forces team in their white Arctic survival suits disembark themselves and their equipment from Wessex XP142 *Humphrey*. (FAA Museum)

Left: Crashed Wessex XT464 lying on its side in the snow on Fortuna Glacier. Fortunately the aircrew and Special Forces team were all rescued with the assistance of Wessex XP142 *Humphrey*. (FAA Museum)

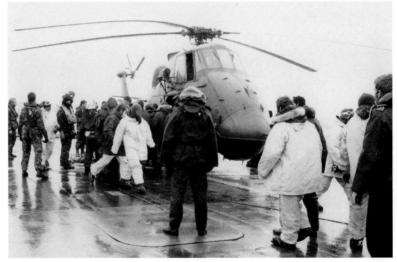

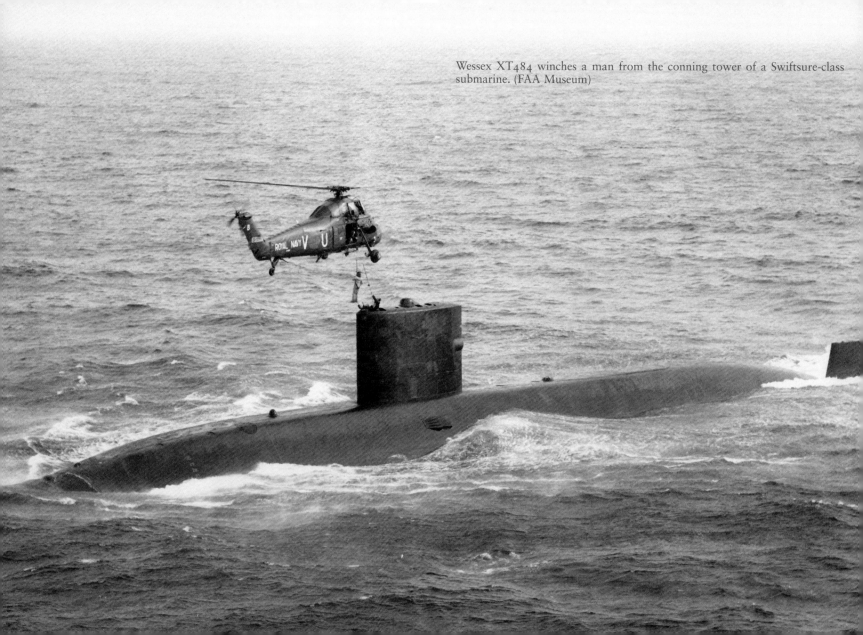

Wessex XT484 winches a man from the conning tower of a Swiftsure-class submarine. (FAA Museum)

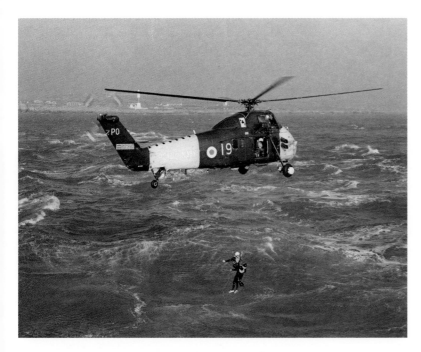

Right: Doing it for real. Wessex XT482 rescues survivors of the yacht *Camargue* during the Fastnet Race in 1979. (FAA Museum)

Left: No. 771 Squadron's Wessex Mk 1 in a winching exercise off Portland Bill. Practising in rough seas and storm conditions develops the essential aircrew skills necessary for live rescue tasks. (FAA Museum)

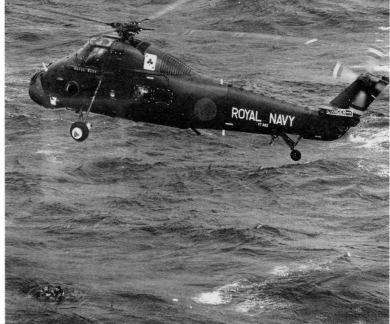

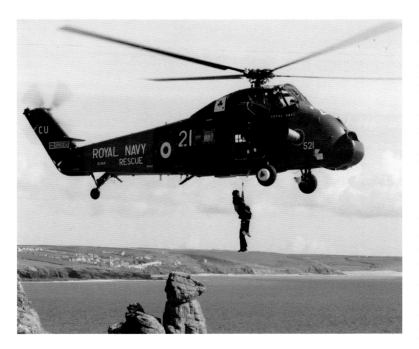

Wessex V seen carrying out a practice lift from a rocky outcrop on the Cornish coast. (FAA Museum)

Having made the tense thirty-mile flight back to HMS *Antrim*, *Humphrey*'s crew unloaded the troops and equipment, refuelled, loaded medical supplies and blankets, and set out immediately back to the glacier to relocate the stricken Wessex 'F'. The weather was still severe and two attempts to get back on to the glacier were abandoned as, even with the onboard radar, it was just not safe to risk the helicopter and crew, no matter how urgent the situation. *Humphrey* headed back to the ship to once more refuel and to await any kind of break in the weather that might allow one successful flight onto the glacier. One small piece of good news during this anxious period of waiting was that radio contact with Wessex 'F' had been established, and confirmed that, miraculously, no one was severely injured. At 1635 hours, as light was fading and the likelihood of making a flight back onto the glacier that day was reducing by the minute, a small break in the weather gave *Humphrey*'s crew the last chance they were hoping for. They set out immediately toward the glacier and quickly located the crashed Wessex, despite the deteriorating weather conditions. Managing to find a reasonably safe landing zone, they landed and squeezed all twelve of the SAS troops and their equipment into the rear cabin of *Humphrey*. Being an anti-submarine aircraft, a great deal of *Humphrey*'s cabin space was occupied with radar, radio and other heavy specialist electrical equipment, so getting twelve men and even more equipment into the back was a difficult task. With the weather closing in again and daylight fading very fast, the very heavily laden *Humphrey* staggered back to HMS *Antrim*, finally managing to bring the last of the survivors from a treacherous mountain operation and two aircraft crashes back to safety.

8

WESTLAND WASP AND LYNX HELICOPTERS

By the late 1950s, Westland Helicopters Ltd were leading the manufacture of British helicopters and beginning to develop their own designs. The Westland Wasp was the result of a design project to create a helicopter that could operate from frigate-sized warships, and was able to carry two homing torpedoes to combat the growing Cold War submarine threat. In addition to its torpedo-carrying role, the Wasp could carry three passengers (plus the crew) or a small under-slung load. One interesting design feature was the incorporation of bulges in the rear cabin doors to accommodate foot and head ends of a stretcher placed within the rear compartment. This additional comfort for a casevac patient responded to the design fault on earlier small-bodied helicopters (e.g. Hoverfly and Dragonfly), where the casualty or rescued party would sometimes have to protrude from the doorway after being picked up.

By the late 1960s Westland Helicopters Ltd began a joint design project with the French-based company Aérospatiale, and from this emerged the replacement to the Wasp, the Westland Lynx. With a range of 400 miles and a maximum in service speed of 144 mph, the Lynx has proved to be an extremely capable helicopter, seeing service with no fewer than fifteen Royal Navy small ships' flights.

Although not primarily designed as search and rescue helicopters, both the Wasp and Lynx have proved themselves many times as being very capable at performing rescues under extreme conditions. In home waters rescue, assistance would normally be carried out by the designated SAR squadrons. However, when difficult circumstances arise in foreign waters, where the only helicopter support available is that of a small ship's flight, then the Wasp and Lynx have often come to the rescue.

One account relayed by Cdr Richard Seymour details an operation that earned him an AFC for his flying skills on Wasp helicopters in the early 1970s:

In June 1972, HMS *Yarmouth* was the Hong Kong guard ship, and had disembarked its Wasp helicopter and the flight personnel to RAF Kai Tak for continuation flying for

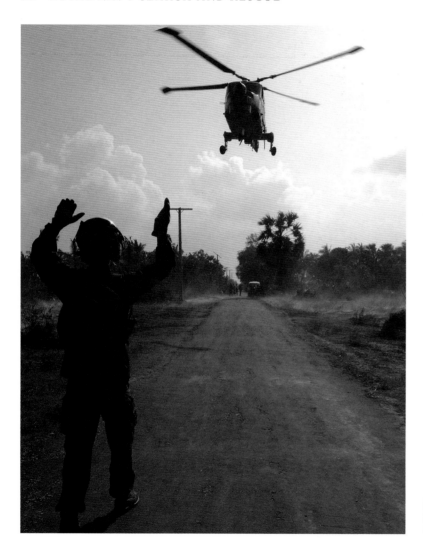

the following month. In early July Hurricane Susan brewing in the South China Sea threatened Hong Kong and as was common practice, all ships sailed to weather the storm at sea. *Yarmouth's* Captain correctly decided that there was no point in embarking the Wasp, and we were better off at Kai Tak. In fact, 'Susan' did not hit Hong Kong and remained offshore.

On 12 July, the Commodore Hong Kong received a signal that a container ship, SS *Oriental Falcon*, had been swept onto the Pratas Reef during the hurricane some 150 miles east and required urgent assistance. *Yarmouth* was tasked to proceed to that area; it was agreed that the Wasp was the only realistic way of any rescue, and that the flight be re-embarked while the ship steamed east. An RAF Wessex was called upon to assist by taking the six flight personnel, and my aircrewman, L. A. Dick Taggart, and I took off in company with the Wessex to join the ship some 80 miles from Hong Kong – clearly a one way trip for the Wasp even on full fuel!

On arrival onboard, it was clear that the Wasp needed to refuel and be relaunched as quickly as possible, to locate the stricken ship before dark. It was decided to take the Assistant Flight Deck Officer, Sub Lt Lippiett, to be winched onboard to coordinate the rescue, and we launched at dusk some 25 miles from the reef.

Medical supplies, fresh water and emergency equipment being delivered by Lynx helicopter as part of the Philippines hurricane relief operation. (MOD Crown Copyright 2014)

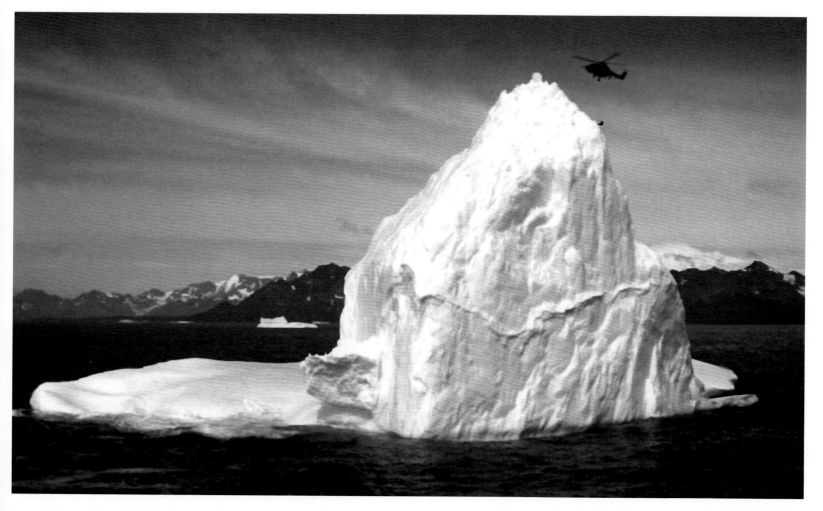

Lynx helicopter from HMS *Endurance* using an iceberg in the Antarctic for winching practice. (MOD Crown Copyright 2014)

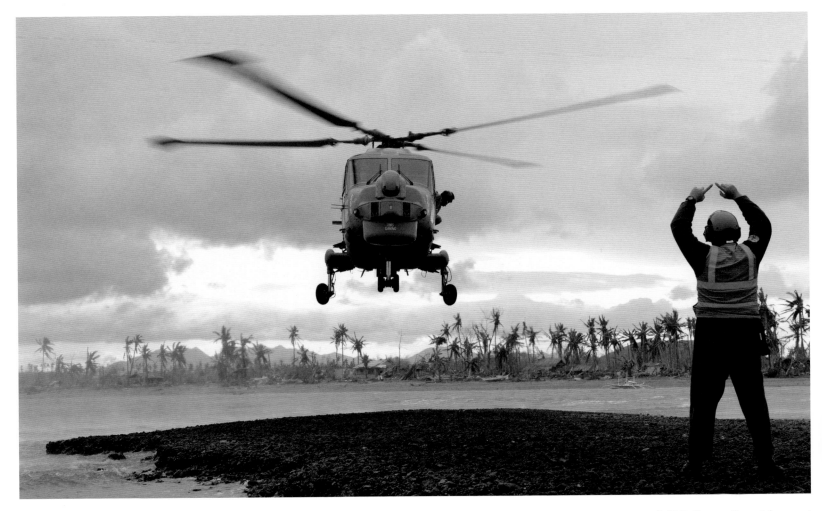

Using any suitable landing zone, a Lynx from HMS *Daring* brings medical teams in to assist with the Hurricane Haiyan emergency. (MOD Crown Copyright 2014)

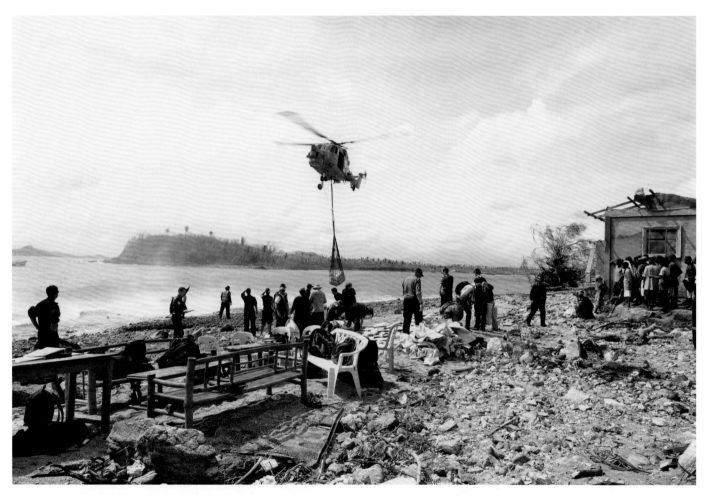

Kalmadu Village, Sri Lanka, in 2004. Royal Navy Lynx helicopters air-lift emergency crews in to assist with the Tsunami relief operation. (MOD Crown Copyright 2014)

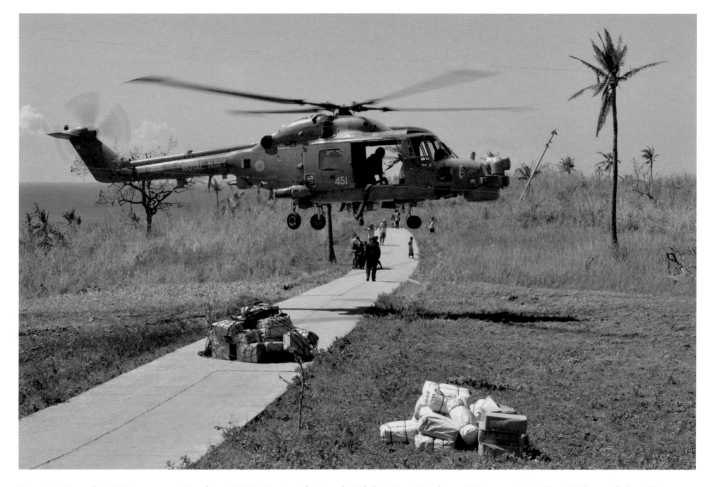

No. 815 Squadron's Lynx operating from HMS *Daring* during the Philippines' Typhoon Haiyan crisis. The children of the villages on Guintacan Island spelt the word 'HELP' on their playground to alert the SAR crew and guide them to their aid with medical supplies. (MOD Crown Copyright 2014)

In fading light we reached the reef and located the *Oriental Falcon*: She was beached broadside on the reef with the wind blowing onto the beam, so positioning to hover just forward of the ship's bridge was satisfactory, using the outline of the superstructure and two of the ship's stump masts as references. Sub Lt Lippiett was winched down to assess the situation and would be the key to liaising with the master of the ship in coordinating the rescue plan. While this was going on, I pulled away from the wreck and orbited close by to conserve fuel. In a very short space of time, Sub Lt Lippiett had managed to rig some temporary lights onto the stump masts and also a few torches suspended on a line between the stump masts which acted as a rudimentary horizon bar. The pick up point was identified as a space in front of the bridge, in what can be best described as a hole surrounded by ship's containers, measuring about twenty five feet by forty, far too small to land in. I had to manoeuvre back into a position over this small dark space and try to maintain a steady hover at about forty feet while we winched some of the crew aboard. Four were winched up singly, but we had now been in the hover for some time, so keeping an eye on our fuel state was a high priority. We pulled away and headed in the direction of where HMS *Yarmouth* would be by now, but had two new problems. Firstly we were not sure of the exact location of HMS *Yarmouth*, and secondly were now experiencing intermittent radio and generator problems: this was probably due to the heavy rain and the fact that it was Standard Operating Procedure (SOP) to fly without doors over the sea (to ease escape in a ditching) and this meant rain swirling around in the cockpit. Very low

on fuel and in total darkness, we again knew that we had to find the ship first time or we could be forced to ditch in a very rough sea, or marginally better, return to the reef and land in the shallow water close to the *Oriental Falcon* – neither an attractive option! To our enormous relief we eventually regained radio contact with *Yarmouth*, and were able to deliver the first few survivors, refuel and return to the reef. We picked up a further nine crew, the ship's Master and

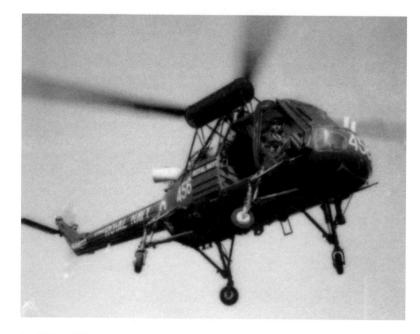

Lt Richard Seymour in the hover over the flight deck of HMS *Yarmouth* in Wasp XT442. (R. Seymour)

the remaining twenty eight crew decided to stay onboard, and after over two hours flying in darkness we landed, and HMS *Yarmouth* returned to Hong Kong so that those rescued could receive medical treatment.

The following day, HMS *Yarmouth* was ordered to return to the reef to pick up the remaining crew, arriving just after four in the afternoon. The weather was still bad, with poor visibility in heavy rain, but we were now familiar with the wreck and how best to position over it. Although very poor weather it was at least daylight and we were able to rescue the remaining twenty nine crew in eight sorties, and around two and half hours flying. HMS *Yarmouth* proceeded to Hong Kong and the survivors from the *Oriental Falcon* were landed the following morning.

Multiple lifts are usually associated with larger helicopters, but Cdr Seymour's modest recounting of events is testament to the capability of this small helicopter in competent hands.

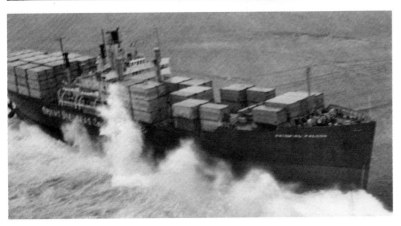

Top left: Log book entry reads simply '*Oriental Falcon* SAR', giving no reference to the difficult and demanding flying that resulted in Lt Seymour being awarded the Air Force Cross. (R. Seymour)

Left: The *Oriental Falcon* aground on the Pratus Reef two days later as the severity of the hurricane was reducing. (R. Seymour)

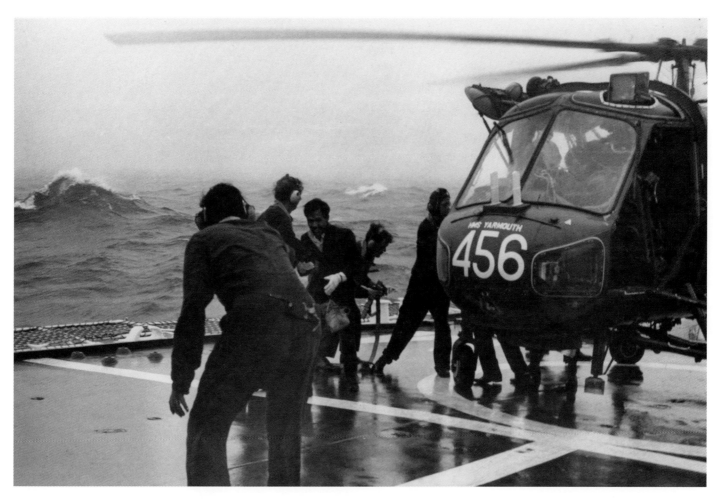

Survivors from the merchant ship *Oriental Falcon* are assisted from Lt Seymour's Wasp helicopter on HMS *Yarmouth*. The angle of the flight deck and the size of the waves in the background give a good indication of the very difficult flying conditions. (R. Seymour)

9

WESTLAND SEA KING

As with a number of Westland Helicopters which have emanated from Sikorsky designs, the Westland Sea King follows that pattern. The first three trials aircraft were delivered to the Yeovil factory in 1967 as Sikorsky S-61B. The Sea King, which developed from these trials, was a huge step forward, providing a helicopter capable of carrying payloads and weapons systems way in excess of that of other helicopters in the Fleet. Its four-hour flight duration would also significantly extend its capability as a submarine hunter-killer and make a vast difference to its ability as an SAR platform.

An entire book could be written about Sea King SAR operations, but one event in particular sums up best of all what SAR training and teamwork culminates in, and is perhaps best relayed first hand in the words of Cdr Mike Norman.

Cdr Mike Norman OBE AFC RN Retd:

The most challenging and dangerous rescue I ever did

I was ashore from the aircraft carrier HMS *Hermes* at Culdrose and as the Senior Observer of 814 Squadron over the Christmas leave period of December/January 1978/79, had responsibility for three Sea King Search and Rescue crews. The weather during that period was very severe with heavy snow, freezing conditions and frequent blizzards. The night of 30th December was particularly bad with severe easterly gales in the Channel gusting to Storm Force 10. My crew was the standby SAR duty crew, the first crew were already airborne on a mission but had made a forced landing in a cabbage field near Marazion, due to atrocious weather.

A Grimsby stern trawler, MV *Ben Asdale*, was tied up alongside a Russian factory ship, the *Antarctika*, anchored in Falmouth Bay and was transferring its catch while attempting to repair a steering gear problem at the same time. In this endeavour the Russian ship had put two of its engineers onboard to assist. However, as the storm conditions worsened the *Antarctika* began to drag her anchor in the heavy seas. At this point the trawler had to be suddenly cast off for the best protection of both vessels,

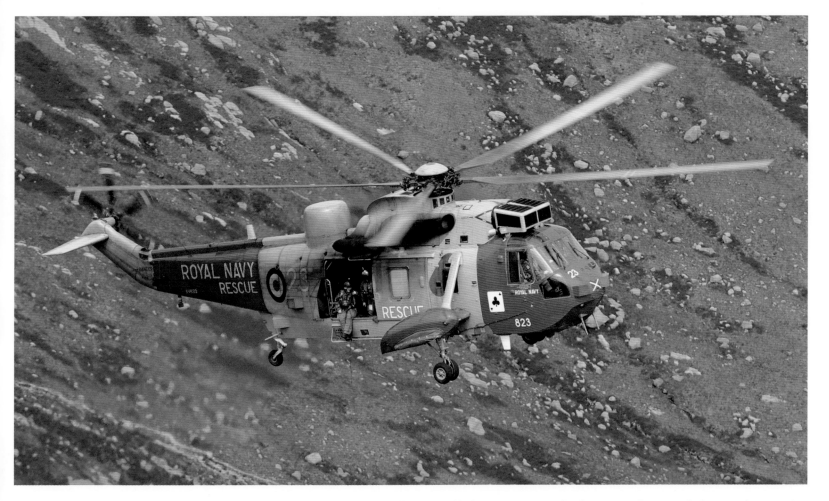

Sea King from HMS *Gannet* on an exercise in the Scottish mountains. The yellow rotor blade serves as a visual indicator to other aircraft that may be operating or passing overhead. (MOD Crown Copyright 2014)

with the two Russian engineers still onboard. There was now a very serious situation with an uncontrollable trawler cast adrift in high seas, now with fourteen people on board. In storm conditions and huge seas the drifting trawler was soon swept into Maenporth Cove and dashed upon the rocks. Conditions were now very violent and the gale force was 9–10 and gusting harder at times. The trawler crew were all in grave danger and had to be rescued as quickly as possible. Responding to their 'Mayday' call the Falmouth Lifeboat was now on scene, but could not get close to the trawler, jammed in the cove.

The Coastguard service by now had a team on the cliffs above the stricken trawler and was attempting to establish a rocket-fired line between the trawler and the cliff top to provide a rescue line. Again the weather was so bad and the seas so rough that the line passed between the trawler and the cliff top soon broke as the trawler rolled over on to its port side. It was at this point (around midnight) that we got a call from the Coastguard. The weather was certainly beyond safe flying conditions and arguably it was not safe to consider sending a helicopter. But there were people in trouble, what do you do? The station Captain, Jock Tofts, was aware of the request and unusually, due to the severity of the storm, came to the operations room during the briefing session to discuss the situation. There were a lot of concerns and reservations about attempting a flight, but then we received another call from the Coastguard informing us that some of the trawler crew were attempting to jump to the rocks. Miraculously, three of the crew had managed to scramble ashore, but three had disappeared.

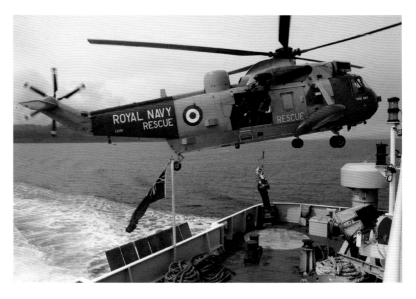

Close winching practice exercise using a Caledonian McBrayne ferry. Hovering this low and close to a moving ship requires great pilot skill. (MOD Crown Copyright 2014)

However, there were still eight people on board and it was clear there was no other means of rescue.

Aware of the considerable risks, the blizzard and the fact that it was pitch black and gusting 50 to 60 miles per hour, we nonetheless decided to attempt a rescue rather than leave the crew to perish on the rocks. We completed our flight preparations and hurriedly gathered together some blankets. We also gained a brave volunteer medic from the Sick Bay who we would certainly need to help with the

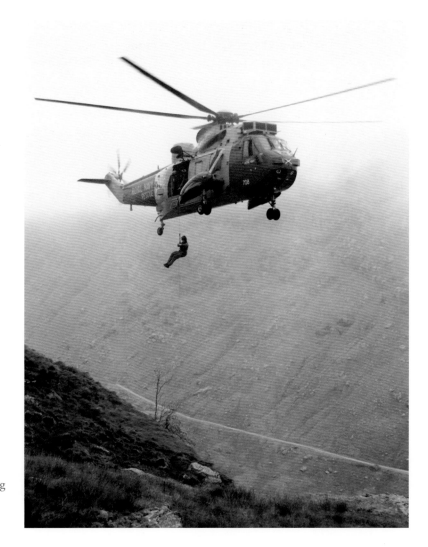

Winching exercise in a Scottish glen with fog and cloud closing in. Operating in mountainous regions is difficult to start with, but when the tops of the mountains become shrouded in cloud or fog, the flying becomes extremely demanding and dangerous. (MOD Crown Copyright 2014)

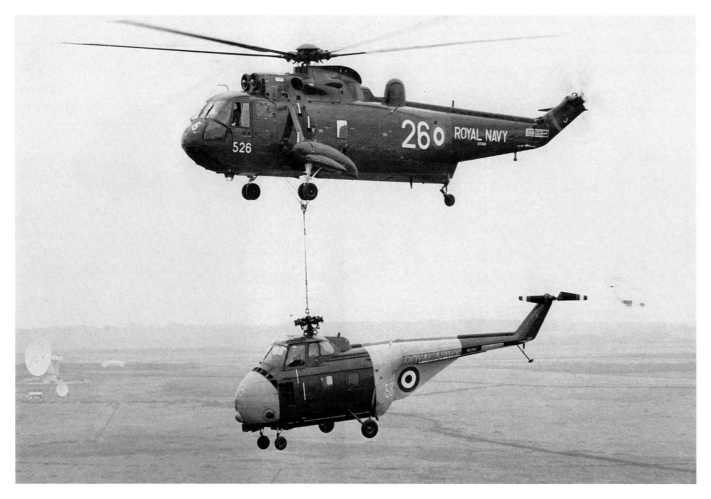

Rescuer rescued! With its rotor blades removed, Whirlwind XN297 is airlifted back to RNAS Culdrose by Sea King XV648 following an emergency landing in a nearby field. (FAA Museum)

survivors. We struggled out into the black night from the warmth of our briefing room, leaning into the wind and blizzard and slipping on the compacted ice and snow. We made it to the aircraft parked on the hard standing. How the ground crew had prepared the aircraft for flight in these conditions, God only knows. The temperature was now at freezing point and this was of major concern. There was a real danger that ice would form in flight and build up in the mouth of the engine intakes, the risk being that lumps of ice could break off and be ingested straight into the engine. Should this happen we could easily have a second catastrophe on our hands. Having carried out pre-take off checks we took off into the black wild night with visibility almost zero. Using the helicopter's radar I was able to navigate the aircraft safely out over the sea, flying at around 200 feet to reduce the risk of icing. The pilots could see nothing so our radar was essential. Putting on our searchlights didn't help much as the beams reflected back off the driving snow. We turned north once clear of the coast at Looe Bar and headed towards Maenporth Cove and the stricken vessel.

During the short turbulent flight we discussed our options and concluded that we would need help from the Coastguard on the cliff top in locating the wreck. We established radio contact with the Coastguard and asked them to shine their search light vertically from their point on the cliff so that we might get a visual reference of their location. Visibility continued to be atrocious. We climbed to 500 feet for safety as we neared the cliffs at Maenporth Cove, and we did get a visual on the Coastguard's light. However, due to the strong easterly gale and eastward facing shoreline we could not descend to the hover from seaward. (Helicopters need to carry out this manoeuvre flying into the wind.) The only option was to overfly the Coastguard's position on the cliff top and head out over the cliffs to the sea, descending as we did so. We accomplished this despite being wildly buffeted by the turbulence close inshore. We established ourselves in a high hover about 1,000 yards offshore and I moved from my radar position to the doorway. What confronted the winchman and I as we opened the sliding door was driving snow and sea spray and huge 30 ft angry seas rolling underneath us, eerily green in our downward facing lights ,and crashing on the shore and cliffs in the blackness behind us. We would have to somehow fly blindly backwards towards the unseen cliffs until we could see the *Ben Asdale*. We asked the Coastguard to give us directions over the radio since they would be able to see our bright flashing lights even though we could no longer see their searchlight. The second pilot took on this task. I took control of the hover trim controller, a small joystick near the cabin door, and started to fly the aircraft rearwards under guidance from the Coastguard while the first pilot kept the aircraft's height at 60 ft. This was a really challenging team effort. Normally under these conditions it would have been considered impossible. But we knew we were the only means of rescue as we slowly inched our way backwards towards the cliffs and the wreck. This seemed to take an eternity but at about 100 yards from the cliffs the second pilot jubilantly reported that he could see the *Ben Asdale* in the Coastguard's searchlight beam, behind us and to our left. We arrived at the scene to see the trawler almost on its side close in under the cliffs and being swamped and battered by the enormous waves rolling over it, slamming it further onto the rocks. Apart from the trawler's stern gantry it almost completely disappeared from view as each successive wave came crashing in. The deafening noise of the huge waves and wind in the confines of the cove appeared to drown out the noise of our own engines, or so it seemed.

There was no time to lose. Through the driving spray and snow we could see one of the crew on the bow of the trawler and looking like he might try and jump for the rocks. We had to go for him first, and very quickly, if we were to stop him from being swept away or jumping to almost certain death.

The problem was getting the helicopter into position to be able to get a winch cable and rescue harness down to him. This was exceptionally dangerous because of the gusting wind conditions, the violent turbulence and the proximity of the unseen cliffs. Judging the position of the cliff face was difficult in the extreme, but somehow we had to do it. Their lives were hanging in the balance. Pulling away now and leaving them to certain death was something that none of us could contemplate. So we came up with a plan. Our training and experience would now really come into play.

The First Pilot, Lt Tony Hogg, had responsibility for flying the aircraft and he would keep the helicopter at the right height using the radio altimeter, while the Second Pilot in the left hand seat and nearest to the cliff face, Lt Larry Jeram-Croft, would direct our own searchlight onto the cliff face and keep our rotor blades at a safe distance while continuing to be the radio link with the Coastguard. I would fly the aircraft over the wreck using the small joystick in the cabin doorway, making the critical fine adjustments to the helicopter's hover position over the wreck. The next decision to make was the type of rescue. Normally I would put the aircrewman down on the deck of the vessel to organise the survivors but under these circumstances that was totally out of the question as I watched the huge waves roll over the vessel, mostly obliterating it from view. So we would have to rescue the survivors by lowering the rescue harness on the winch hook, to a position where the survivors could grab it and put it around their bodies. This was the winchman's job, Leading Aircrewman Chris Folland, and required a lot of skill to ensure that the winch cable and hook did not get snagged on any part of the vessel. If we had had to use the explosive cable cutter to free ourselves it would be 'game over' since we only had one rescue winch. The margin for error under such extreme conditions was tiny but as dangerous as it was, we began the rescue.

I manoeuvred the aircraft over the man on the trawler's bow, keeping up a running commentary on the intercom as to what was happening below us while Chris Folland lowered the wildly gyrating rescue harness down to the man on the trawler's bow and hoped that he would work out how to put it on. Of course, he would not have been trained in how to pass the harness over his head and under his armpits and the fact that he was terrified and suffering from hypothermia did nothing to aid the situation or his thinking. At the third attempt we got it close enough to him and he made a desperate leap and grabbed the harness. He

WESTLAND SEA KING   111

was now hanging to the harness with both hands like his life depended on it, which of course it did. I indicated to the winchman to winch him up fast! – and hope for the best. There was no other option. If he lost his strength or his hold on the harness he would be gone. Miraculously we got him up and into the cabin before he let go. He was very wet and looked bewildered and terrified from his ordeal. We handed him over to the medic, Brian Steele, but he had very little in the way of medical equipment as we had left base in a hurry and with no time to assemble more kit. Thankfully we had a few warm blankets, but not much else.

With one on board, we had no time to lose. We took stock of the situation. OK so far we all agreed, but there were still seven more men to rescue. I manoeuvred the aircraft back over the wreck again while the Second Pilot continued to watch the cliff face. The rest of the survivors were all sheltering in the wheelhouse. We had to judge when to lower the harness as the seas continued to swamp the vessel. Chris Folland would take some slack winch wire and drop it the last few feet when the time was right. Between us we managed to get the harness down to the next man who had appeared outside the wheelhouse. He made a grab for the harness and this time the survivor did know how to put it over his head and under his armpits and tighten down on the toggle for a snug fit. This lift went fairly smoothly and we now had two safely aboard. The trouble now was that we were running out of space in the cabin. This was a specialist anti-submarine helicopter and as such had a lot of submarine hunting equipment such as sonar in the cabin. There was very little room for survivors. I discussed

the situation with Tony Hogg and we agreed that I would manoeuvre the aircraft clear of the vessel and hand back control to him while we reorganised ourselves in the cabin. We would have to move the survivors forward, up a narrow passage to a seating area in front of the sonar winch. This we managed to do which also helped the aircraft's centre of gravity. We had been hovering increasingly tail down.

For the third lift we decided that the First Pilot would retain full control of the aircraft while I passed verbal directions over the intercom; for example 'Come forward and left 10 feet'. The trouble is, there is an inherent delay in this. By the time the pilot has moved the aircraft to the new position the situation below us has already changed, especially in such violent conditions. That is why the aircraft is fitted with a flight control joystick in the doorway, to cut out this communication delay. However, despite all the best communication efforts between the pilots and myself on the intercom, it was difficult to keep the aircraft on station over the wreck and the survivor. We were being wildly buffeted by the gale force winds and the first pilot was having trouble controlling the aircraft while responding to my directions. Consequently we were not directly overhead the survivor when we lifted him clear, the result being that a huge 'swing' developed. As he wildly spun and swung around under the helicopter, the winch cable became snagged around a piece of the aircraft structure behind the cabin doorway. This was very serious indeed. The steel cable was now sawing into the aircraft structure as we continued to reel in the winch. Folland stopped the winch and bravely reaching outside and behind tried to free the cable, but this proved impossible. We could not now winch the man into the cabin. The only way to free the line was to lower the man down and take the weight off the cable. Putting him back on the trawler was not an option, nor was flying him back to Culdrose, hanging below the aircraft. He would be frozen stiff and dead before we got there. That would also mean terminating the rescue and leaving the remaining crew to their fate. In a split second we decided that the only option was to hover out to sea, clear of the cliffs and lower the survivor into the huge seas which would take the weight off the winch cable, enabling Folland to free it. So this is what we did; what the survivor thought we were doing God only knows. With the man now in the freezing sea, Folland, who was 6 ft 4 inches tall, was able to lean out of the doorway and free the cable from its obstruction. That done we quickly gained height and winched the bedraggled and very cold man on board. He was suffering from hypothermia without doubt.

With no time to lose and with the pilots keeping a close eye on our fuel situation (we had been airborne about an hour and a half), we had to repeat our rearward transit into the cove under radio guidance from the Coastguard. (What would we have done without them?) At this point they informed us that during the last lift when we had difficulty controlling the aircraft, our rotor blades had come within inches of the cliff face. At this point, as Captain of the aircraft, I seriously thought about abandoning the rest of the survivors to their fate. We had a discussion about the options and concluded that we just had to try our utmost even though all safety considerations told us otherwise.

With five survivors still to be rescued I took control of the hover control joystick once again, not wanting to repeat the near disaster of the last lift. One by one we picked the men off the trawler, but by the time we were down to the last two or three we were experiencing internal communication problems. The winchman and I had spent most of the time hanging out of the cabin doorway in the teeth of the gale and had not noticed that our helmets and visors were caked in snow and ice. The snow and spray from the waves had played havoc with our microphones, and communication between us was now very intermittent. We performed the last two rescues with no radio communication at all, using hand signals and passing scribbled notes between myself and the pilots. This took valuable time and used up precious fuel, but it was the only way we could complete the rescue. Fuel was now a major concern because we had been hovering in violent turbulent conditions with large fluctuating demands for power being made on the engines. Also we had no means of knowing if there was a build up of ice in the engine intakes.

With the last man onboard and with a cabin now crammed full of very cold hypothermic survivors who needed urgent medical treatment, our priority was to return to base as quickly as possible. We returned to our crew seats and a quick look at the radar screen enabled me to scribble one more note to the pilots 'Climb to 500 ft and turn south'. As we climbed away from the cove, the pilots were able to establish some sort of radio contact with the airfield. We had been out of contact for over three hours but they had been kept informed of the progress by the Coastguard. Just when we thought the worst was over we were informed that there had been a complete power failure on the grid and that the airfield emergency generators were providing sufficient power for communications only, but no airfield radar. The wind was now gusting Storm Force 10 or more in a continuing heavy blizzard and freezing conditions. It was still pitch black night and visibility was zero and we still had a difficult task ahead to find our way home. We headed south along the coast at about 200 feet using the aircraft's radar picture which was very 'cluttered' due to the rough seas. As we neared the airbase we climbed to 500 ft for safety. We could see nothing below but blackness. When I was as sure as I could be that we were overhead the centre of the airfield and clear of obstructions, Tony established the aircraft in a high hover and commenced a slow vertical descent in the swirling snow and blackness while I sat there hoping that we were where I thought we were. We descended slowly and blindly until at about 50 feet on the altimeter the second pilot caught sight of the ground in our lights. What a relief! In swirling snow we touched

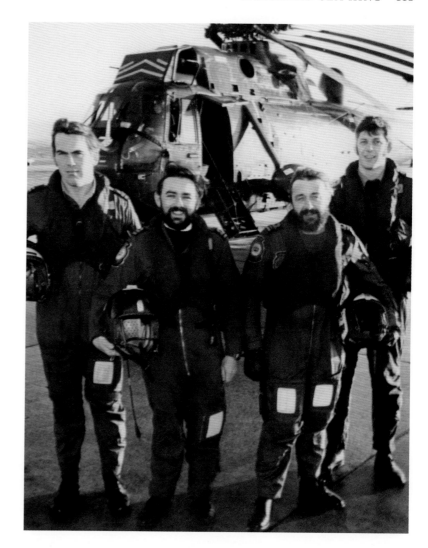

The crew of Sea King 592 after the *Ben Asdale* rescue. From left to right: Pilot Lt Tony Hogg (awarded AFC); Second Pilot Lt Larry Jerram-Croft (Queen's Commendation for Valuable Service in the Air); Lt Commander Mike Norman (awarded AFC); Leading Aircrewman Jan Folland (Queen's Commendation for Valuable Service in the Air). Missing from the line up is Leading Medical Assistant Brian Steele, who was not normally a member of this aircraft crew, but who volunteered his services on the night of the 31 December 1978. He received the Queen's Commendation for Brave Conduct. (Mike Norman)

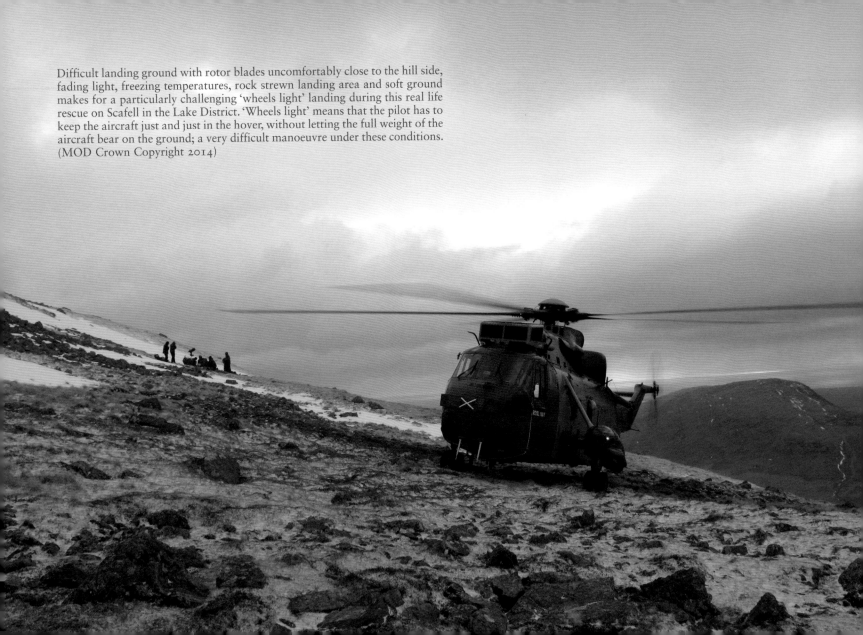

Difficult landing ground with rotor blades uncomfortably close to the hill side, fading light, freezing temperatures, rock strewn landing area and soft ground makes for a particularly challenging 'wheels light' landing during this real life rescue on Scafell in the Lake District. 'Wheels light' means that the pilot has to keep the aircraft just and just in the hover, without letting the full weight of the aircraft bear on the ground; a very difficult manoeuvre under these conditions. (MOD Crown Copyright 2014)

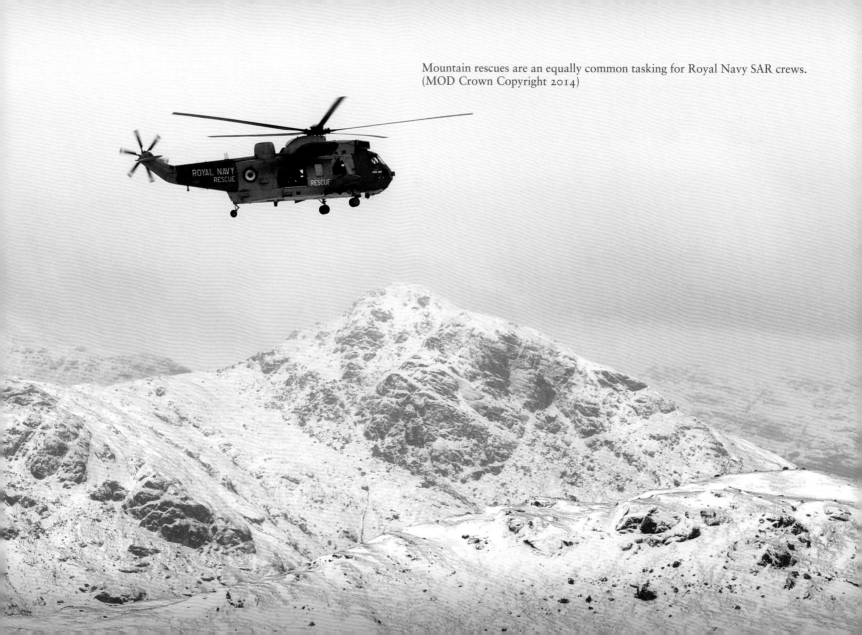

Mountain rescues are an equally common tasking for Royal Navy SAR crews. (MOD Crown Copyright 2014)

down on the compacted snow and ice. We had done it. The ambulance was ready and waiting to collect the survivors, so we shut down the aircraft without further delay and helped the medics get them into the ambulance.

The ground was covered in packed snow and it took quite some time to get the aircraft safely back into the hangar, with the towing tractor slipping and slithering all over the place. We all had to lend a hand pushing and shoving our 15-ton aircraft inside, which had performed brilliantly over the last few hours.

With the aircraft undergoing post-flight servicing, we got out of our wet flying kit and had a well earned cup of coffee. About an hour or so later we went down to the medical centre to check on the rescued trawler men and to see how they were. I made a point of meeting the one surviving Russian engineer and the skipper, Barty Coe, who expressed their collective gratitude for what we had done, especially as he had been told by someone that we didn't have to fly the mission in view of the appalling weather. They were clearly very grateful for the fact that we had saved their lives, but it was sad to reflect that three had not made it. (We were to learn the next day that their bodies were washed up on the beach; one of them was one of the two Russian engineers who had volunteered to help the *Ben Asdale*).

It was now about 7.00 a.m. and starting to get light and we could now see the blizzard and gale force winds and wondered how we had managed to fly safely in such conditions. We had not slept since yesterday and were looking forward to a bit of 'shuteye' in the crewroom.

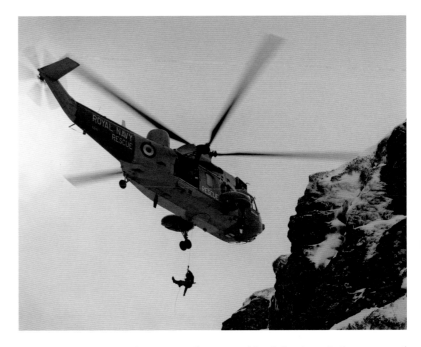

Practice, practice, practice – you only get good by doing it, as is demonstrated in this high mountain winching exercise. (MOD Crown Copyright 2014)

However, right then the phone rang. It was the Operations Room informing us that a woman had gone into labour and urgently needed to be air lifted to hospital as the surrounding roads were still impassable …

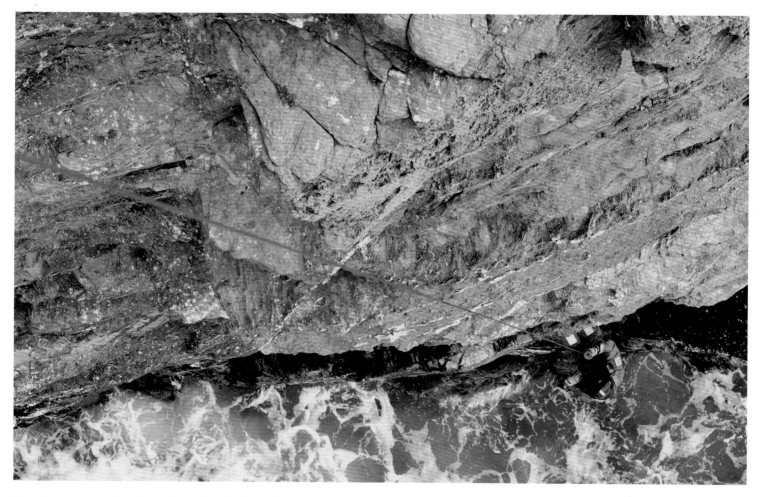

The aircrewman's safety is now in the hands of the pilot, positioning him close to the cliff to deal with a situation or stranded person. (MOD Crown Copyright 2014)

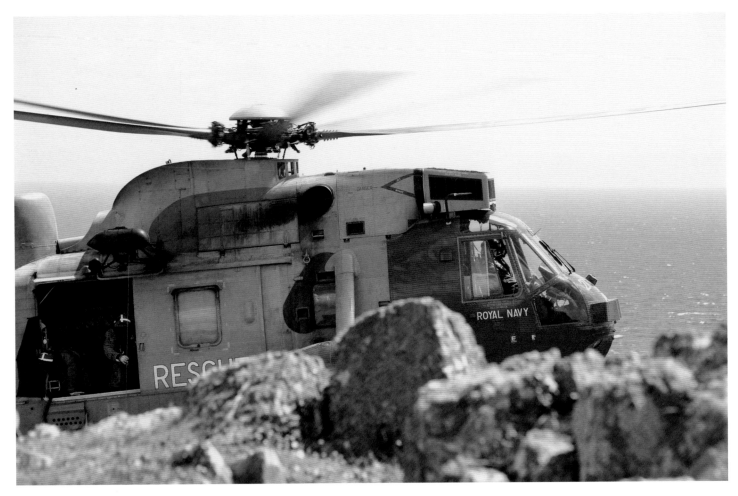

Close cliff winch training is still an essential SAR exercise that keeps the whole crew trained and familiar with this potentially very dangerous task. Keeping the helicopter in position very close to a cliff face demands immense concentration and flying skill. (MOD Crown Copyright 2014)

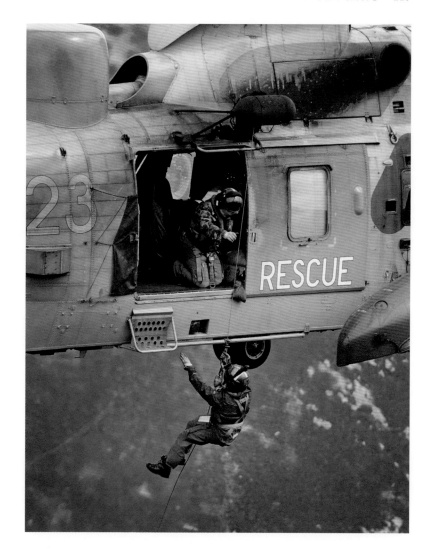

Sea King crew from HMS *Gannet* prepare to begin a mountain winching exercise. (MOD Crown Copyright 2014)

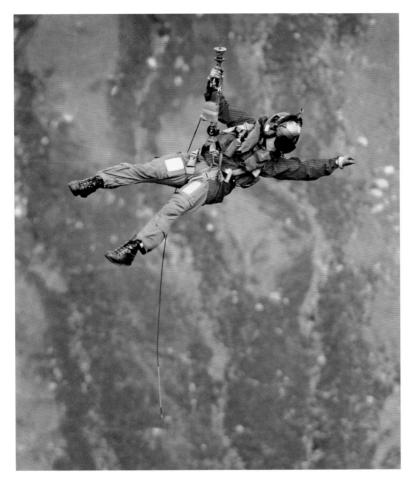

Girl on a wire: Lt Angela Webb shows that today this is a job for the girls as well as the boys, if you have a head for heights! (MOD Crown Copyright 2014)

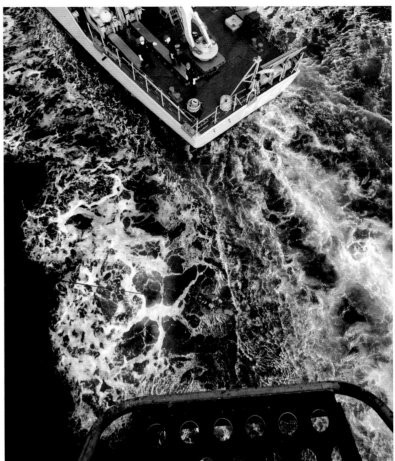

Winching exercise from the winch operator's viewpoint. Gauging height and position of the aircrewman/diver requires a lot of practice to place him safely in position. (MOD Crown Copyright 2014)

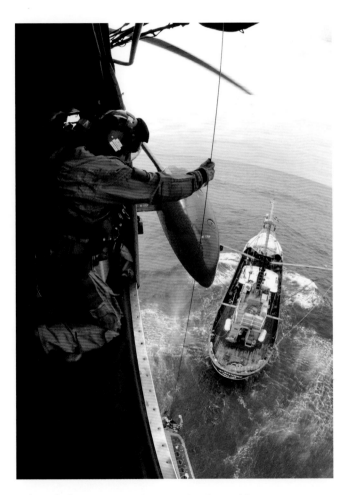

What all the training is for – getting in position to recover an injured fisherman from a trawler off the Cornish coast. (MOD Crown Copyright 2014)

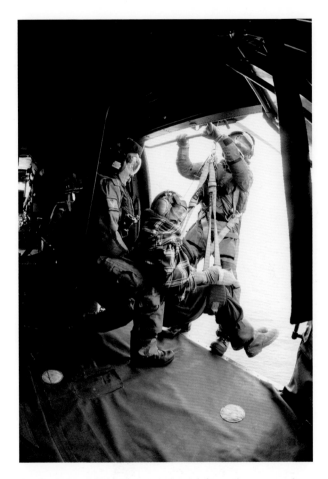

As the injured fisherman is released from the rescue sling, the aircrewman braces himself across the door to prevent the fisherman falling from the helicopter as the harness is disconnected. (MOD Crown Copyright 2014)

10

EH101 – MERLIN

As the Sea King bows out after forty-six years in Royal Navy service, the mighty Agusta-Westland Merlin EH101 takes over as the new generation of highly versatile anti-submarine, general utility and battlefield support helicopters. Navy helicopter aircrew will continue to be trained in SAR duties for service requirements. However, from 2016 the Royal Navy will hand responsibility for civilian SAR (and other public emergency responses that require an aircraft) over to the Coast Guard and other airborne emergency services, thus bringing to a close a service that has seen many civilian lives saved during the last 100 years.

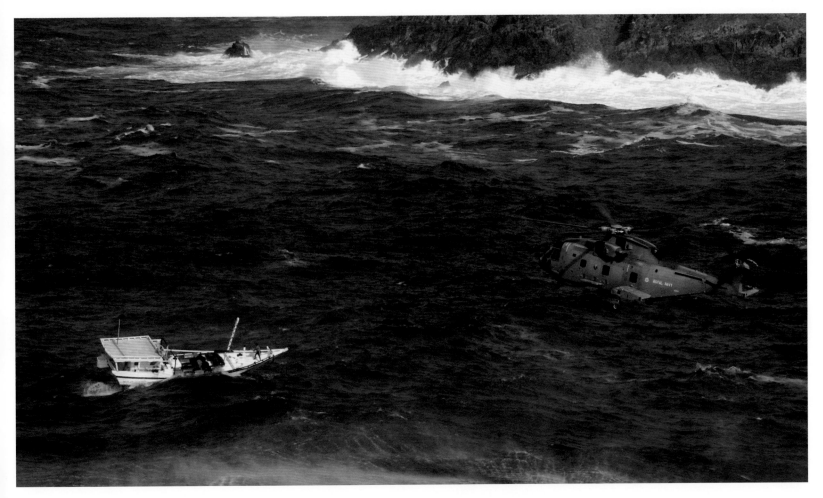

A Royal Navy Merlin helicopter from HMS *Illustrious* rescues fisherman from a stricken vessel off the coast of Somalia during a Storm Force 7 gale. (MOD Crown Copyright 2014)

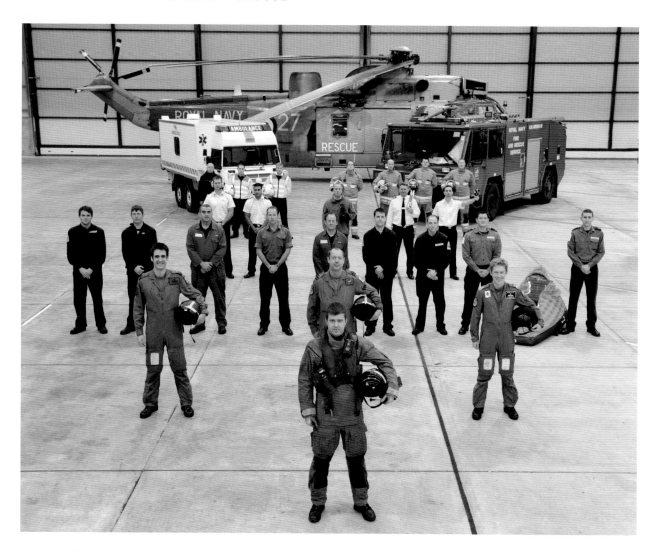

Team work: pilot, observer, aircrew, engineers, survival equipment teams, emergency services and medical staff are all an essential part of the SAR team. (MOD Crown Copyright 2014)

ACKNOWLEDGEMENTS

With grateful thanks to former Royal Navy helicopter squadron maintainer Jerry Shore, whose assistance and additional knowledge through previous close association with Royal Naval Search and Rescue squadrons has been extremely valuable.

Fleet Air Arm Museum, Barbara Gilbert, Jonathan Coombes, Thomas Langham, Catherine Cooper, Robert Turner, Mike Burrow, Lee Howard. Royal Navy UK Regions Media, Fiona Holland, Emma Relton RN PRO Culdrose. Steve Saywell, RN Fleet Photographic Unit Editor. Capt. E. M. Brown RN CBE DSC AFC, Capt. M. J. F. Rawlinson RN OBE. Cdr R. P. Seymour RN AFC, Lt Graham Foster RN, Cdr M. Norman RN OBE AFC. Surg. Cdr R. T. Jolly RN OBE.

RAF Museum, Hendon. Mansfield Spong. Alan Beattie, Steve Hague, Yorkshire Helicopter Preservation Group. J. Waldron-Jodies' Jungle Jaunts.com, Sarawak Tourism Board, Rudi Anoi. Cornish Photos. Denis Jory.

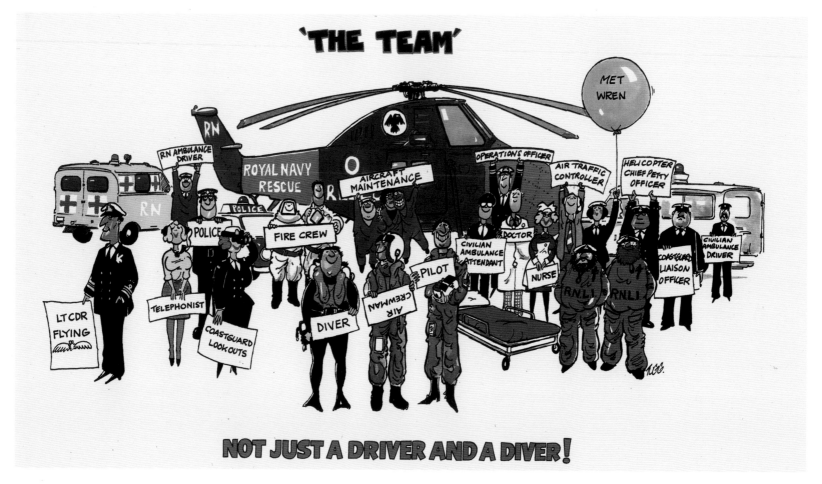

Using humour to make a message remain memorable, few people have ever had the talent of Navy Cartoonist Lt Cecil 'Tugg' Wilson. His SAR poster 'The Team – Not Just a Driver and a Diver' is typical of his ability to capture the character and behaviour of individuals and service units alike. (MOD Crown Copyright 2014)

BIBLIOGRAPHY

Owen Thetford, *Royal Naval Aircraft Since 1912*, (Putnam Aeronautical Books: Sixth revised Edition, 1991)

Ray Sturtivant and Theo Balance, *The Squadrons of the Fleet Air Arm*, (Air Britain Publication, 1994)

C. F. Snowden-Gamble, *The Story of a North Sea Air Station*, (Oxford University Press, 1928)

George V. Galdorisi and Thomas Phillips, *Leave No Man Behind: The Saga of Combat Search and Rescue*, (Motorbooks International, 2007)

Aeroplane Journal, 1919.

John Winton, *For Those in Peril*, (Hale Press, London)

Various Pilot's Log Books, Squadron Record books, Line Books and Diaries from the Fleet Air Arm Museum Research Centre.